PRAISE FOR
SARAH RAYNER'S NOVELS

'*Brilliant... Warm and approachable.*' **Essentials**

'*Carefully crafted and empathetic.*' **Sunday Times**

'*A sympathetic insight into the causes and effects of mental ill-health as it affects ordinary people. Powerful.*' **My Weekly**

'*Explores an emotive subject with great sensitivity.*' **Sunday Express**

'*Delicious, big hearted, utterly addictive... irresistible.*' **Marie Claire**

'*Rayner's characters ring true, their concerns are realistic and their emotions guileless. Ripe for filming, this novel is both poignant and authentic.*' **Kirkus Reviews**

'*Rayner's delicate, compassionate exploration of the struggles women face with fertility will resonate loud and clear with anyone struggling to have a family.*' **Publishers Weekly**

ABOUT THE AUTHORS

Dr Patrick Fitzgerald
MB.BS MRCGP Diploma in Palliative Medicine

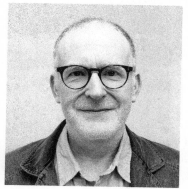

Patrick is a General Practitioner and hospice doctor working in Cheshire. He studied medicine in London and became a GP in 2007. He has a special interest in cancer and palliative care and has worked as a GP educator for Macmillan Cancer Care, in hospices and with community and hospital palliative care teams.

Sarah Rayner

Sarah Rayner is the author of five novels including the international bestseller, *One Moment, One Morning*[1]. In 2014 she published *Making Friends with Anxiety, a warm, supportive little book to help ease worry and panic.* This was followed by a series of books including *Making Friends with the Menopause* and *Making Friends with Depression* which she co-authored with

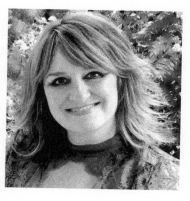

Dr Patrick Fitzgerald. In 2017 Sarah set up the small press, **creativepumpkinpublishing.com** and *Making Peace with the End of Life* is one of the imprint's launch titles.

Sarah lives in Brighton with her husband, Tom, and you can find her on Facebook, Twitter and Instagram via her website, **sarah-rayner.com**.

NON-FICTION BY SARAH RAYNER
Making Friends: A series of warm, supportive guides to help you on life's journey

Making Friends with Anxiety:
A warm, supportive little book to help ease worry and panic

More Making Friends with Anxiety:
A little book of creative activities to help reduce stress and worries

BY SARAH RAYNER AND DR PATRICK FITZGERALD
Making Friends with the Menopause:
A clear and comforting guide to support you as your body changes

BY SARAH RAYNER, KATE HARRISON AND DR PATRICK FITZGERALD
Making Friends with Depression:
A warm and wise companion to recovery

BY SARAH RAYNER AND PIA PASTERNACK
Making Peace with Divorce:
A warm, supportive guide to separating and starting anew

BY SARAH RAYNER AND TRACEY SAINSBURY
Making Friends with your Fertility:
A clear and comforting guide to reproductive health

BY SARAH RAYNER AND JULES MILLER
Making Friends with Anxiety:
A Calming Colouring Book

NOVELS BY SARAH RAYNER

Another Night, Another Day
The Two Week Wait
One Moment, One Morning
Getting Even
The Other Half

DR PATRICK FITZGERALD
SARAH RAYNER

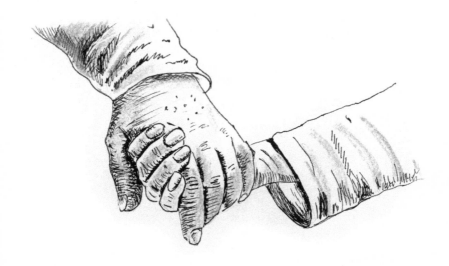

Making Peace
with the
End of Life

A clear and comforting guide
to help you live well to the last

Featuring illustrations by Sarah Rayner

This edition first published in 2017 by Creative Pumpkin Publishing, an imprint of The Creative Pumpkin Ltd., 5 Howard Terrace, Brighton, East Sussex, BN1 3TR.

www.creativepumpkinpublishing.com

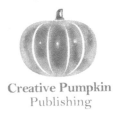

Creative Pumpkin
Publishing

First Edition October 2017
ISBN: 9780995794832

Cover design and illustrations: © Sarah Rayner.

Publisher's Note:

Making Peace with the End of Life provides information on a wide range of health and medical matters, but is not intended as a substitute for professional diagnosis. Any person with a condition or symptoms requiring medical attention should consult a fully qualified practitioner. While the advice and information in the book are believed to be accurate and true at the time of going to press, neither of the authors can accept any legal responsibility or liability for any errors or omissions that may have been made, nor for any inaccuracies nor for any loss, harm or injury that comes from following instructions or advice in this book.

HELLO AND WELCOME

Making Peace with the End of Life is here to keep you company on the journey from diagnosis through the weeks and months ahead, to the last days of life. It can't stop what's coming, but we hope it will make your circumstances a little easier, more comprehensible, and perhaps give moments of peace.

Maybe you've been having treatment for cancer, and have recently been told the disease appears to have spread. Perhaps you have Motor Neurone Disease and it is progressing. Or perhaps you've just turned 75, 80 or even 90, and are experiencing a number of symptoms associated with growing older, and want to be prepared for your future years. It could be that your spouse – or your mum or dad – is in the last stages of Alzheimer's. Or it's possible that you're a carer or health worker responsible for someone with a very serious illness. No matter what your reasons for wanting to learn more, *Making Peace with End of Life* is here to help.

We aim to support and reassure by looking at how you might care for yourself physically and emotionally. We look at how symptoms brought on by life-limiting illnesses can be controlled. We will direct you to supportive services. And of course, this book is about dying, the thing we don't want and can't stop. It's also about legacy, and the memory you leave behind.

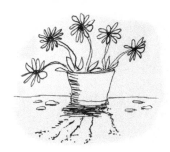

Making Peace with the End of Life is packed full of practical advice, important contact information you may need, alongside fictionalised patient stories to illustrate these often difficult situations. It also aims to demystify how the NHS and Social Services work. Perhaps most importantly, we look at how communicating your wishes to those involved in your care can give a feeling of safety and control over whatever happens in the future.

About me, Dr Patrick Fitzgerald

I'm Patrick Fitzgerald, a GP and hospice doctor, and I've written this book because I want to help improve people's experiences in the last months, weeks and days of their life. It's my job to work within a team that supports those living with life-limiting diseases, which means I have to give difficult news to patients about the diagnosis and the potential future they face. Male or female, young or old, rich or poor and no matter what the specific medical situation, people are rarely prepared or ready to hear what I am going to say. All too often their loved ones are as taken aback as the patient.

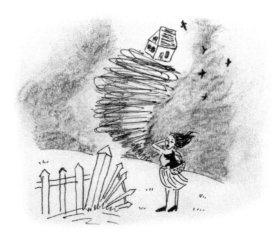

'It can't be true. It just can't be true. It can't be happening to me!'
Debbie, 55

Helping you and those who care for you

When you're reeling from news like this, there can be too much shock to think clearly about the ramifications, let alone plan accordingly. How on earth can you grasp how the systems work, where to get advice or think clearly about your legacy when you're overwhelmed by what you've just heard? On top of this, the courses of our illnesses can't be accurately predicted: we are individual from our beginning to our ending. Trying to work out how much time lies ahead is fraught with miscalculation and occasionally inappropriate optimism. I often hear patients talk as if they have five years ahead, when it seems to me more likely as their general practitioner to be only a few months.

In addition, many people feel it has become increasingly difficult to die in the way they would wish. The treatment path can appear complex and confusing, and my sincere hope with this book is to provide some clarity around diagnosis, treatment options including palliative care, and to also look at how we die. By looking at this path, my hope is that this book will bring insight and understanding into how we can approach the end of our lives.

Making Peace with the End of Life is directed towards those who have been told they are now living with a life-shortening illness, so that much of it is written in the second person, 'you', because it's your wellbeing that lies at its heart. However, when we're feeling ill, it can be hard to take in information, so you might like to read what you can, and skip bits that seem overwhelming – you can always come back to them, or avoid them altogether. Everything is clearly signposted and cross-referenced as much as we could manage, and I hope you find what you need. As well as for you, this book is also written for your loved ones and friends and carers, so that they can understand what may lie ahead. You may like to dip into it when you are together, or read bits on your hopes and dreams (in Chapter 2) or your legacy (Chapter 12) and then talk about them. I also hope it helps those who are experiencing the effects of ageing, and want to better understand what may lie ahead as well as get their affairs in order. Healthcare professionals and counsellors might also find it helpful. In short, **it's for *everyone* wanting to know more about end-of-life care and decisions, and the physical and emotional impact of terminal illness.**

We are all different in our needs, and there are no right or wrong ways to read this. **But however you use *Making Peace with the End of Life*, I hope you'll find it like a knowledgeable and compassionate 'friend' who can help you understand what's happening and to support you.**

Talking of friends, this seems a good point to introduce my book-writing companion: Sarah Rayner.

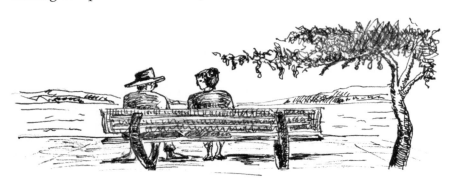

About Sarah Rayner

Sarah and I met 25 years ago in London. For a while we were virtually next-door-neighbours. 'We used to be able to nip round to one another's for a quick cuppa to offload our worries or arrange an evening of Scrabble at a moment's notice,' Sarah remembers. Now we live a couple of hundred miles apart – I'm in the Peak District and she's in Brighton. These days Sarah is a bestselling author – you may know her from *One Moment, One Morning*, or the other books in the *Making Friends* series – and we're still close friends. We've collaborated on two books before – *Making Friends with Depression* and *Making Friends with the Menopause*. 'The series aims to provide clear and comforting guidance on those mental and physical health issues many people find hard to talk about,' says Sarah. Like me, Sarah believes there is a desperate need for concise, clear information to help those at the end of life.

'I don't have Patrick's medical training,' she explains, 'and that's why I was keen for him to write this book. However I do have a lay-woman's experience of caring for people nearing the end of life: when my stepfather, Adrian, was in the last stages of cancer a few years ago, I went to stay in the house with my mum to help care for him, and I was with him when he died, peacefully, at home. My father, Eric, passed away in 2016, after living with Alzheimer's for over a decade. And now I am helping my mum, who is 83 and increasingly vulnerable, with day-to-day care. I've drawn on these experiences to contribute in terms of edits, as well as adding my own specific words and illustrations.'

More about this book

If *Making Peace with the End of Life* was an accurate reflection of what it's like to live with a terminal illness, I'd throw the whole thing in the air and piece it together at random, because that's what I see – a mixed up time made up of sense and confusion. But that wouldn't be much of help to you, so instead it is in a careful order, travelling from mortality and prognosis, through areas of treatment and the law, right to the last few days of life and the weird empty time for those left behind afterwards.

Together Sarah and I are going to try to demystify some of the process ahead and support you and your nearest and dearest at this difficult time. The themes are generalised for all conditions, as my clinical practice has shown me that the process of dying is not absolutely related to a particular illness, but rather there are similarities that we all go through. There is a diagnosis, there are changes, deterioration occurs such as weight loss and fatigue, and this develops over time until we become more and more frail. As others have been where you are, and both Sarah and I have travelled some of the way with them, this means that, in spite of the shock and uncertainty, perhaps there *are* things that can be put into place to make the time ahead a little easier.

There are quite a few books on the end of life, so why read this one in particular?

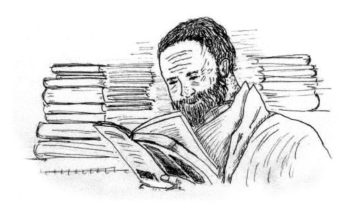

1. Hopefully the pages ahead will empower you to live fully the life and times you have ahead, however brief. We can't change the nature of the news you've been given. We'll explore common worries, such as controlling symptoms of pain and sickness, how to get help staying at home, accessing social care, benefits and debt advice, and how you can best care for yourself and get support from the wonderful providers out there.

2. We know some ways that may make the journey easier and would like to pass them on. No matter if you're just beginning to notice your body changing or are right in the middle of this changing process, *Making Peace with the End of Life* aims to help you work out the best way through. **You'll notice that we've given you check lists and spaces to make notes, so you can use this book as a place to jot things down and work things out.** Keep it to hand and then all your important thoughts and musings will be safe.

3. We won't make false promises. Or offer false hope. *Making Peace with the End of Life* isn't going to fix all your worries and fears as it can't be specific to your case. We aim to be honest about the different situations people face – including ones that are tricky and may be difficult to read about. There is no intention to be unkind or cause alarm – quite the opposite. We'll gently lead you through each subject step by step, in the hope that understanding the changes you're going through may make the process less daunting.

4. Neither Sarah nor I are affiliated to any one doctrine or spiritual practice. Whilst I am a medic, I'm well aware that there are some aspects of my patients' wellbeing that are better handled by counsellors or spiritual guides, and I would be the first to encourage you to seek support from a variety of sources.

5. The idea of life after death is beyond the remit of this book. There are other books by great (and some not so great!) thinkers that tackle this subject. Here, however, **we're concerned with what is happening to you now, and to plan for what might be coming next.**

6. No two people are alike, but it can help to know that you are not alone in going through this experience. With this in mind, we have included examples of conversations with patients with different diseases, at different stages of the process. **Please note that the patient examples in this book are fictionalised, based on an amalgamation of common experiences that Patrick has seen.** Any relation to a true event is purely accidental and unintended.

7. *Making Peace with the End of Life* **is relatively concise.** By the time you've finished, you'll have a good overview. You'll find TIPS, which are emphasised **in bold, like this,** and are designed to give nuggets of advice to help ease your journey, and FACTS, which appear in grey boxes, and aim to give clarity on key points.

8. Please dip into this guide as and when you need to. Whilst some people may be keen to read it from start to finish and digest every word, we appreciate that others may not. **We aim to answer the questions most patients want to ask, but that doesn't mean every question will be relevant to you, or of interest.** You may not feel up to reading some sections at all. **Feel free to focus on specific sections and skim passages, especially when we have included more detail, such as in Chapter 3 (Reaching Out, which is about where to go for help) and Chapter 8 (Medical Treatments, which explores the drugs and interventions you might encounter).**

9. The purpose of this book is to give you access to as much seinformation as possible, without swamping you with text. If you are reading on an electronic device then you should be able to click on the links and open them directly. If you are reading the paperback, then **please note that all of the websites are located at the end of the book.** There is also a bibliography at the end of the book for further information and reading – a wealth of wisdom and great writing from experts in this field.

Patrick and Sarah

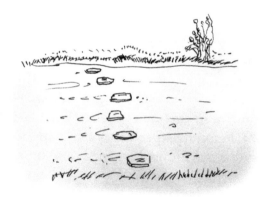

CONTENTS

I. DIAGNOSIS

1. Discovering Your Own Mortality
Yes, we've always known, but to be told this may be your last illness can be a shock and hard to process.
- Ageing
- How our experience of death has changed over time
- Dealing with the immediate stress of diagnosis
  - Asking the right questions
  - Asking more questions
- For your own notes

2. Prognosis – Trying To Predict The Future
Predicting the future is complex, so let's find out how it's done, and why knowledge can be empowering.
- Getting a better sense of your own situation
  - Diagnosis
  - Prognosis
- Working with your prognosis
  - Treatment options – deciding what you want in terms of medical care
    - > EXAMPLE 1
    - > EXAMPLE 2
  - Planning options – your hopes and dreams for the time you have left
    - > OPTION 1 – written notes
    - > OPTION 2 – an advance care plan or statement
- A quick recap
- For your own notes

II. BEING CARED FOR

3. Reaching Out For Help From Your Family And Friends
Who is around to help you? How can they best support you at this difficult time?
- Support from your family and friends
- Communicating with your loved ones
  - A note about boundaries
- Asking for help
- Friends and neighbours
- Care for those who are caring for you
  - Tips for relatives and friends

4. Help From Your Healthcare Teams
A guide to who does what in the clinical support teams, to help you find the care you need.
- Your GP and the Primary Care Team
  - Tips for dealing with your GP
- Nurses – who's who?
  - District Nurse and Macmillan Nurses
  - Other Specialist Nurses
- Your Consultant and the Hospital Team
  - EXAMPLE 1
  - EXAMPLE 2
  - Transport to and from the hospital
- Your Palliative Care Team
  - Allied healthcare professionals
- Hospices
  - What's the difference between a hospice, a care home and a nursing home?
- Getting help and support from charities
- Getting help in an emergency

5. Help For You At Home From Social Services

Finding your way through Social Services can be a confusing business, so here's a helping hand.

- Being assessed by Social Services
  - Assessing your care needs
  - Assessing your finances
  - What sort of help might you get?
  - EXAMPLE 1

  Practical adaptations to make being at home easier
  - EXAMPLE 2
- Co-ordinating care at home
  - EXAMPLE 3
- For your own notes

III. CARING FOR YOURSELF

6. Your Physical Wellbeing

Some simple ways you can look after your own body when you're unwell.

- Food
- Fluids
- Exercise
  - EXAMPLE 1
- Intimacy and sex
- Fatigue
- Vaccination
- Physical changes during illness
- When things get more difficult

7. Your Psychological And Spiritual Wellbeing

Looking after your mind when you're unwell.

- Grieving an illness
- Getting specialist help
  - Assessing mood
  - Talking to a therapist or counsellor

- Where to find a therapist or counsellor
- Medication
- Complementary therapies
- Books that may help
- Spiritual Support
- Coping with work
- Holidays – taking a break from treatment
- Creating hope

IV. TREATMENTS

8. Medical Treatments
What medical teams can offer to control illnesses.
- Options in cancer
  - Surgery
  - Chemotherapy
  - Radiotherapy
- Options in heart failure
  - EXAMPLE 1
- Options in COPD
  - EXAMPLE 2
- Options in neurological disease
  - EXAMPLE 3
- Options in dementia
- Other disease groups
- Some general medical aids explained

9. Aches And Pains – Symptom Management
Trying to ease the symptoms of living with your disease.
- Pain
  - Assessing pain
  - Analgesics
  - Fears about using drugs
  - EXAMPLE 1
  - Adjuvants

- Non-steroidal Anti-Inflammatory Drugs
- Steroids
- Nerve pain or neuropathic pain agents
- Sickness and loss of appetite
- Constipation and diarrhoea
  - EXAMPLE 2
- Breathlessness
- Skin health
- Further complications
  - EXAMPLE 3
- For your own notes

V. PLANNING FOR THE FUTURE

10. The Law

Understanding how the law works, and using it to support your future decisions.

- Making a will
- Capacity and the Mental Capacity Act
  - EXAMPLE 1
- Lasting Power of Attorney (LPA)
  - LPA for Property and Finance
  - LPA for Health
- Advance Decision to Refuse Treatment (ADRT) / A Living Will
- Do Not Attempt Cardiopulmonary Resuscitation (DNACPR)
- Work and the law
  - Fit notes (formerly sick notes)
  - Self-employment
  - Dismissal
- Debt
- Gifts of Money
- Benefits to which you may be entitled
- Other grants

VI. THE ENDING

11. End of Life
Understanding the last days and hours of life
- What usually happens when we die
- Treating physical symptoms in the last days and hours of life
  - EXAMPLE 1
- Where we choose to die
- Unexpected endings – a note for family members
  - EXAMPLE 2
- For your own notes

12. Your Legacy
Your story, in words and pictures, something to leave behind for loved ones.
- Memory boxes and life stories
- Planning a funeral
- Traditional or alternative?
- Financing a funeral
- Memorials

VII. FOR THOSE LEFT BEHIND

13. And Afterwards
- Immediately after death
- Post-mortems and the Coroner
- Registration of death
- Paying the bills
- Probate
- As the days pass
- Last words

Acknowledgements
Endnotes
Charity Contact Details and Useful Websites
Recommended reading – books and articles
Books by Sarah Rayner

- *Making Friends with Anxiety*
- *Making Friends with Depression*
- *Making Friends with the Menopause*
- *Making Friends with Your Fertility*
- *Making Peace with Divorce*
- *One Moment, One Morning*
- *The Two Week Wait*
- *Another Night, Another Day*

I. DIAGNOSIS

1. DISCOVERING YOUR OWN MORTALITY

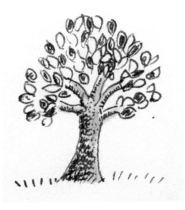

'Why me? Why now? It shouldn't have happened like this? I'm too young – I've got so much more I want to do!' **Joe, 39**

'I remember saying to my husband: "But we've got a holiday booked and a new grandchild on the way – I can't die before then!"' **Petra, 71**

'If heaven will extend my life by ten years more…'
Hokusai, Japanese painter, 90

When I was a child, two things were a shock to me. The first was that my parents weren't supreme beings, that they could be wrong. The second was that they were going to die. I felt worry for the first time, as if my life had lost its moorings. Over time it then dawned on me that I was also going to die. I had no understanding of this at a young age. I couldn't imagine it, not even after attending my first funeral. Until you've been given this news, it's likely that your own mortality was something you knew about in theory, but maybe never quite believed. Death was at some point in the future, distant and vague.

Even if you've been ill for a long time, there is never the right moment to focus on the end of our own life; we tend to defer such difficult thoughts. It's so hard to get your head around the fact that your doctor has told you that whilst medical intervention may delay things, this is likely to be your final illness. You are going to die. Probably not that soon, but still too soon, too soon by far. Your thoughts can run riot, your mind whirling with possibilities: *What will happen now? Can I be cured? What if there isn't a cure? What about my family, my children, my house, my job, my money, my pet, myself?* Hopefully this book will reduce the spin of this merry-go-round, bringing a little peace into the storm.

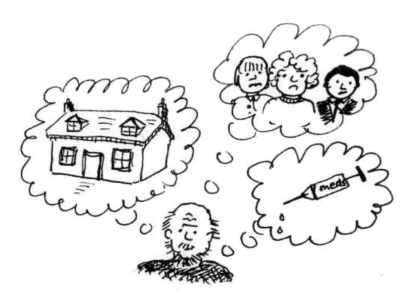

One of the strongest emotions we have is a fear of dying. People have searched over the years for cures to prolong life, for elixirs to regain youth. The sad but inevitable truth is that we are finite; death comes regardless. The ancient Egyptians spent much of their lives preparing for the afterlife, building elaborate funerary rites and burial chambers. Many religions focus on life after death too. You may well have a faith which you can call upon to help you at this time, you may not. What we have to say here in this book doesn't run counter to either stance. Instead, **we're going to concentrate on the things we can do in life to better prepare ourselves for the life we have left to live.**

'What is it like to die?' This is one of the questions my patients often ask me, and we'll look at the process of dying in more detail in Chapter 8. If you're concerned about what might happen, you may find it comforting to dip into that now, as **my experience is that for most patients, dying is a simpler, more gentle process than we might picture in our anxious minds.**

'When my father was very ill, he told one of the carers who was looking after him: "I want to go to sleep now. I want to sleep for a very long time. I want to sleep forever." He died two days later, peacefully. In the morning he'd been disturbed by coughing, but in the afternoon, he calmed, and at some point just drifted off, with my stepmother by his bedside. She says it was so gradual, she wasn't actually sure of the moment when he passed away. She had to listen to see if he was still breathing, and eventually was certain that he wasn't. Later, when I heard what he'd said to his carer, I found it very reassuring: he'd told someone that he was ready. He wanted to go, and that is what he did.' **Sarah**

'My mum had a rough ride from the time of her diagnosis until we got her into the hospice. The hospital where she had her surgery made her agitated and depressed. Once she got to the hospice she seemed to settle. She was there for 10 days, mostly in bed, but with a constant flow of friends keeping her company. I was holding her hand when she died, and it was so quiet. Even though I had seen death numerous times, I had to get the nurse to make sure that it had happened. I couldn't quite believe how peaceful it had been.' **Patrick**

1.1 Ageing

One of the other questions my patients tend to ask me is: *'Why is death inevitable?'* Let's continue by looking at the natural ageing of the cells in our bodies. **All of our cells are programmed to replicate and then, in time, to perish.** It's a natural cycle: we are born, we reproduce, we age, we die. It's the same for every living creature and in an abstract way this is fine, until it happens to us. As human beings, there seems to be an overestimation of our ability to survive. Whilst perhaps it would be wise to be more aware of our mortality and start planning before something happens, all too often we don't. Maybe that's how we can continue to get out of bed in the morning, work at jobs we don't fully enjoy, while away hours doing things we're not interested in or put off conversations we know we should have – because we believe tomorrow is coming and that there is still time ahead to be lived. It's almost as if we're programmed to believe ourselves immortal. Tomorrow probably *is* coming, but one day it won't, and, facing the full force of this is almost always a shock and feels unfair. **We'll look more at the psychological impact of learning that you are nearing the end of life in Chapter 7, and give you some pointers on how to take care of your mental health at this difficult time, and where you might seek support.**

1.2 How our experience of death has changed over time

This sense of unreality is perhaps compounded because dying has become less visible to us than it was to our ancestors. A hundred years ago it was a familiar experience: women dying in childbirth was common, as was death in childhood. If you lived to forty, you were doing well. Today, with improvements in public health, sanitation and vaccination, we can expect to live much longer, with an average life expectancy of around eighty for men, and a little more for women[2].

Not only has life expectancy improved, but it has become less common for people to die at home. Instead, death occurs more commonly in hospital and care homes, with the process more medicalised and the end of life seeming less of a natural and acceptable process that follows growing old. Dying has become a more abstract prospect, with doctors offering more interventions and treatment.

The result is that nowadays death can be a stranger to us, something distant, even taboo. Most of us rarely talk about it until we're forced to, perhaps only when someone close to us becomes seriously ill. Just think of all the euphemisms surrounding the subject: we talk of someone 'passing away', 'being no longer with us' and 'resting in peace', and we joke about them 'kicking the bucket'. Making light of it makes it less of an issue, perhaps.

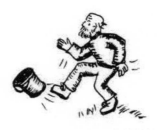

If the *age* we die has changed and *where* we die has changed, it's also worth reminding ourselves that what we die *from* has also changed. Years ago infection was the commonest cause of death: you were more likely to die of tuberculosis or influenza, for instance[3]. The most common cause of death in the UK today is heart disease. We now live longer and die from different conditions from 100 years ago.

Despite these changes in the common causes of death, there remains huge variety in what we die from. Our bodies fail in ways that are as individual as we are. As we age our bodies stiffen, behave out of character, and eventually wear out, leading to diseases like kidney failure, heart failure and dementia. Abnormal cells that used to be picked off by our immune system are instead allowed to grow, with cancers then developing. While many of these diseases can bring about a slow deterioration, sometimes decline can be rapid or hard to predict – for example, a stroke or heart attack can take us quickly.

On top of our bodies failing there are the unexpected accidents of life: falls, car crashes, drowning. These unpredictable events cause huge upset, with no time to plan or prepare, with loved ones left behind, suddenly bereft. (You might like to have a look at our book, *Making Friends With Depression*, if this situation is pertinent to you.)

Whatever diagnosis has been given to us, it is a time of reassessment because things have now changed.

1.3 Dealing with the immediate stress of diagnosis

When we are given a serious diagnosis, one that suggests that time ahead is shortened or less than expected, we can lose our bearings. As the world turns upside down and uncertainty whirls around us, questions and fears abound, mostly associated with *what lies ahead.*

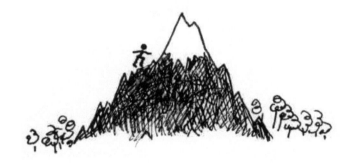

'Where do I start? My head is all over the place! Do I tell the kids? Do I quit work? Do I just give up? Do I try to climb Mount Everest?? I have no idea what to do.' **Jenny, 55**

Firstly, this isn't a time to make decisions. Shock means lots of adrenalin is pumping around, making you worried and anxious. It's likely that you're not thinking clearly. Beware of unexpected impulses to do something new. They can be hazardous. A desire to spend money quickly or to take an extravagant holiday may be rash for instance.

22

TIP: Don't decide anything yet. Give yourself time to digest the information – a week or two if you can. Allow your feelings to settle and the waves of shock to pass. Insight will come gradually, both from discussions with your medical teams and also by sharing your fears and worries with your loved ones. They will help you to make some sense at this seemingly senseless time.

We're all such different creatures with different needs that also vary from day to day. If you have a young family, your worries may be very different from those of someone in their 90s. If you live on your own, your experience will not be the same as it is for someone living within a large family, and it may well be harder to cope. If you already suffer from depression or anxiety, it's extremely natural for these feelings to be greatly heightened when you receive a diagnosis. If this sounds like you, it's well worth watching out for any worsening – you and/or your loved ones can find pointers in Chapter 7.

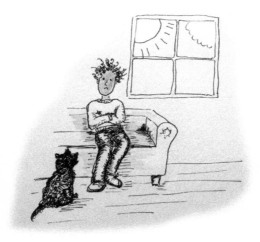

TIP: Try not to keep the diagnosis to yourself. Your loved ones are there to support you. It's unlikely that divulging information will upset them any more than it has upset you. They may have questions too, but be assured they are very likely to want the best for you. 'Protecting' someone from your secret may only end up isolating you from each other.

1.3i Asking the right questions

TIP: When your head is all over the place, making a list of questions for your doctor can help to organise your thoughts. You may like to do this with someone else – a partner if you have one, or a family member or close friend – as two minds are often better than one.

Perhaps consider the questions below, where we've left space for you (or a friend) to write notes. **You may also like to ask someone to come with you to your appointments. It's often easier to talk together afterwards and clarify what was said.**

- **Do you fully understand what the doctor told you?** Shock can make your memory unreliable. Do you need to make another appointment to go through the diagnosis again?

  Write your question here: ....

- **What information do you need?** Is there something specific, such as treatment side effects? Has the doctor used medical terminology that is difficult to understand?

  ....

  ....

- **Do you have questions about the disease itself?** e.g. are you concerned about it being contagious? Are you unsure as to how the disease progresses?

  ....

- **Does this diagnosis impact on other long-term conditions you might have?** If you suffer from rheumatoid arthritis, for instance.

  ....

- **Do you have questions about what happens next?** Are you clear about what options are available? Your doctor may have already discussed these, but you may have been deaf to all that was said as your mind clouded over with too much information.

....

....

- **Where will treatment take place?** Perhaps your lack of fitness concerns you: will you be able to get there? Will you be well enough?

....

- **What do you do about your holiday that you've just booked?**

....

- **How much time can you have off work?**

....

- **What should you tell your family?**

....

....

- **Are the doctors absolutely sure about this diagnosis?**

....

....

Your doctor may not have all the answers, but hopefully they can point you in the right direction of where to get further support.

1.3ii Asking more questions

As time goes on, your need for information will probably change. Here's a second list to consider, and please add your own questions specific to your situation:

- **What are you most concerned about?**

  ....

- **Are you worrying about pain?**

  ....

- **Are you worrying about how your appearance may change** e.g. hair loss, weight loss, taste changes?

  ....

- **Are you worrying about the process of dying?**

  ....

- **Are you thinking about who's left behind?**

  ....

- **Are you thinking about what happens after you die?** In particular, is there a religious concern?

  ....

- **Are you worrying about your house?**

  ....

- **About money?**

....

What else? Write it down here. Don't underestimate the small things such as: 'Will I still be able to meet my walking group every Tuesday?', 'Can I still pick up my grandchild from school?' and 'Will I see next Christmas?'

....

....

....

TIP: Be wary of the internet: it may give more information, but it can trigger anxiety. Bad news tends to make the headlines, not nice reassuring stories – and yet there *are* reassuring stories, as Sarah's description of her father's death shows.

So now we've looked at some of the questions you might be asking to help you get a clearer picture as to what is happening, let's take a look at what the future might hold, and explore some of the issues around a prognosis.

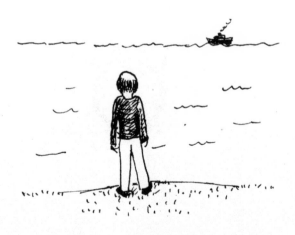

For your own notes:

....

....

....

....

....

....

....

....

....

....

....

....

....

....

....

....

2. PROGNOSIS
TRYING TO PREDICT THE FUTURE

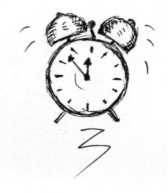

'I can't think of anything. Everything is fuzzy, like a headache. I keep going to work like nothing is happening, waiting for my chemo date. This is crazy, just crazy.' **Danny 54**

'I'd like to know what treatments are available, but I don't want to know how much time they might "buy" me.' **Jenny, 28**

'I want my oncologist to be plain with me. Tell me what the scans show.' **Des, 63**

After delivering bad news to my patients, one of the first questions I tend to get asked is *'How long have I got?'* **But before you ask that question of your doctor, consider how much you would like to know.** Some are hungry for all the information they can get. Others are the opposite, finding that not knowing the details of their treatment or illness makes it easier to cope.

TIP: Doctors can sometimes give you too much information, or news that you don't want. It's a good idea to let them know your limits, sometimes called 'boundaries'. There's more advice on setting boundaries in Chapter 4.

2.1 Getting a better sense of your own situation

Whilst I have sympathy with those who choose not to know, I do believe it is worth getting an idea of your prognosis, as **there are things that you can do with this information. It allows you to plan, make decisions and, decide on the things that are most important to you.** If I repeat this as we go along it's because I feel it is central to making sure you live well with whatever time lies ahead.

2.1i Diagnosis

Back to the question: *how much time have I got?* It's a fair thing to ask, but in truth no doctor – me included – knows the exact answer. Your GP – as the name 'General Practitioner' suggests – will in all likelihood have had a generalist training, so they will make informed guesses, by watching trends, seeing how things change and comparing this to experiences they have had with other patients. Even if an honest answer might be *'Less time than you would imagine, and far less time than you would like'*, that's a hard thing to say and even harder to hear. An accurate diagnosis[4] can help to gauge not only what time may lie ahead, but also work out what treatment options are available. However not all diagnoses are straightforward:

- **Some diagnoses can be clear** – a breast lump that turns out to be cancerous, and on CT scanning the cancer appears to have spread. This is called *metastatic disease* – the cancer has spread from the original organ to elsewhere in the body. The diagnosis is metastatic breast cancer.

- **Some diagnoses are harder to gauge** – the extent of heart failure is determined by a combination of breathlessness, fluid accumulation, chest pain and the ability to do activity, for instance. These symptoms can vary over time. With medication and bed-rest, a patient can change from sudden deterioration to miraculously returning to a state of previous weeks. This can be deceptive though; the trend is one of deterioration all the same.

2.1ii Prognosis

FACT: No one ever knows exactly when they are going to die.

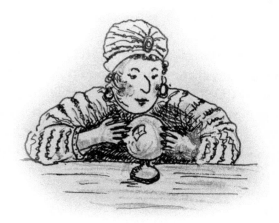

Instead, what clinicians can offer is a *prognosis*, a prediction about the course of a disease. A helpful way of looking at what might happen in the coming months, weeks and days is by drawing upon the methods of the Gold Standards Framework (GSF) charity team[5]. It was put together for medical teams to improve the experiences of patients at the end of their lives, from improving control of symptoms to ensuring that as much planning has been put in place as possible. In order to help GPs to better support patients living with a life-limiting disease, the GSF team encourages medics like me to try and predict who in our care might have six to 12 months left to live, and to discuss their cases frequently. We are aware that sometimes our patients can die quickly or suddenly; there are accidents, heart attacks and strokes, which we can't anticipate. What the Gold Standards Framework proposes is that **those with cancer, those with deteriorating long-term conditions like heart failure, and those with dementia tend to follow patterns that are, at least to some extent, predictable.**

These are only generalizations and, being such, the exceptions to these predictions are many, but let's look at these prognoses in the broad brush strokes that the GSF team proposes:

- **For cancer patients a diagnosis is made and, if there is widespread incurable disease, then decline tends to be continuous, without pause.** The speed of decline will depend on the type and severity of the cancer. Some cancers can be very aggressive, others less so.
- **For those with deteriorating long-term conditions, like heart failure and chronic obstructive pulmonary disease, (often called COPD), it's less predictable.** Sudden events can happen which suggest that time is short, but then recuperation occurs. It's like a swing, going back and forth, recovery and deterioration, recovery then deterioration, but the trend is worsening function, as the pendulum loses momentum and the recoveries lessen.
- **Dementia sees patients drifting downward more slowly, muddling along, as thinking, mobility and understanding lessen and lessen.** Frailty increases, with potential falls, accompanied by reduced appetite and intake. This 'slippery slope' tends to be shallow and gentle.

As with all predictions, there are wide variations in experience. Why is it so difficult to predict what will happen, and why can it be so wrong at times? The answer to this is that statistics tell us one story but the individual tells their own unique version. Some patients with cancer, particularly elderly patients, can rally because the cancer is slow in its destructive work. Advances in chemotherapy have also altered our expectations, with new immunotherapies providing more optimistic outcomes.

'At eighty, my stepfather was given one to two years to live, and told that with chemotherapy it was more likely to be two. At first I thought he looked unlikely to last 18 months – the chemo walloped him so hard. But in fact he lived for three years and only in the last three months did he seriously deteriorate.' **Sarah**

Patients with heart failure can have sudden events and so, as I've touched upon, can die more quickly than a generalised prediction would suggest. Equally some dementia patients, particularly younger ones, can deteriorate quickly, almost as if they have a cancer. Those with neurological disorders – like Motor Neurone Disease (MND) or Parkinson's Disease, for instance – can have experiences that are hugely different from one another, in spite of being diagnosed with the same disease.

But what about you? Am I saying there's *no* knowing? **Hospital doctors are more specialised than GPs, and thus more familiar with their disease groups, which usually gives them a better feel for what the future might look like.** They can show you statistics that look at averages of survival. An oncologist might talk of one-year and five-year survival rates, with the numbers dropping over time. An oncologist might say 'Patients with lung cancer that has already metastasised tend to have a poor outlook'. Still, how does an insight like this help you? You're a person, not a number. Yes, you may eventually form part of these statistics – as might we all – but you're not a statistic in yourself. **Your GP will in all likelihood have known you the longest and be better placed to assess changes in your condition.**

TIP: The combination of your GP and hospital consultant predictions should give you a clearer picture.

There's one other consideration, and that's that conditions change as time passes, and this gives clinicians the strongest clues as to what is happening. Your medical team will be following you up, and this will mean they are better able to make educated guesses over the weeks and months ahead. My common phrase to patients at the hospice is: *'I'll know more about how things are going, the longer I know you'*. Watching changes happen gives us insight as we see and sense losses: a dropped cup, getting stuck in a chair or the bath, a fall, weight loss. We notice increasing tiredness, reduced appetite and food intake, and more time spent in bed resting. This is accompanied by a decreasing ability to look after oneself, with more reliance on others. All of this alerts us to a shortening of time left ahead.

2.2 Working with your prognosis

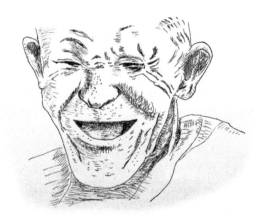

2.2i Treatment options – deciding what you want in terms of medical care

Whilst a diagnosis alone may be a trigger for anxiety and sorrow (something we'll return to in Chapter 4) and any prognosis is a grey area, **knowledge can be empowering.** Whilst we can't predict for sure how your disease is going to play out, thinking about what is important to you may help you move from panic and helplessness to a place of feeling more in control. I don't say this lightly; **considering what matters to you can help you and your medical team determine the value of any treatments on offer, helping you balance the risk and side effects of intervention, versus the time you would like to, perhaps, spend travelling or with your loved ones.**

TIP: Ask yourself: what do I want from any treatment offered? Will I take the treatment regardless of how it will make me feel, or do I want to try it and see how I go? If I don't want treatment now, can they offer it to me later? What will happen if I decide not to have any treatment?

These are big and important questions. The answer is unlikely to come in a flash, and we've given you some space to write down your thoughts here:

....

....

....

....

....

....

....

....

TIP: Don't make a snap decision. Give yourself time. Chat through things with your loved ones. If you're trying to work your way through this alone, then the old adage *sleep on it* **can be useful.**

Once you have a clearer picture of what you'd like, you can discuss these things with your medical team. You might want to ask them:

- If treatment will interfere with specific plans you have. With chemotherapy, for example, you may feel unwell for a while but then have more quality time ahead. But it may be the exact opposite. Often it's possible to work around important commitments.
- Will the side effects and time spent at hospital have a positive outcome – in other words, will it help you feel well enough to do the things you enjoy?
- Will treatment return you to feeling better, as well as living longer?

Here's a space to write down what you want to ask your medical team:

....

....

....

....

....

....

....

....

....

> **FACT: It may not be straightforward to talk through treatment options without also talking about your prognosis, so please bear this in mind when you work out your questions.**

When considering treatment options, **it's important to acknowledge that each of us is different in our ability to tolerate information, medication and a hospital environment.** Let me illustrate.

EXAMPLE 1

Chronic obstructive pulmonary disease (COPD) is a term that covers a wide range of lung disease. It is characterised by deteriorating airways function, mostly due to stiffening and inflammation of the lung tissue.

Let's meet my patient Kenny, who has severe COPD. Kenny lives close to his nephew, Ian. He also has a dog, Lucy, who he is very fond of. Kenny is on oxygen most of the time and he takes Morphine a couple of times a day for his breathlessness, which helps, but it makes him constipated so he doesn't like using it much. Kenny still has the odd cigarette when he turns off his oxygen. It matters to him that he can still do this, even though he is so frail. It also matters that he can get to the shops with his portable oxygen.

Kenny and I have talked things through. He knows that he is very ill and his lungs could give out at any point. Some months ago we had a few difficult conversations to better understand what was important to Kenny. Together we decided:

- To avoid hospital admissions we would treat chest infections at home whenever possible.
- Kenny would try to get someone to help look after Lucy as it was becoming too much effort for him to look after her.
- Kenny would turn off his oxygen if he smoked, as it is a fire hazard and he needed his oxygen to feel well. Tricky as he could have had it taken away by the fire department! But he stuck to this promise.

- Kenny would give Power of Attorney for his health and finances to his nephew Ian, in case he couldn't make decisions in the future. I directed him to Age UK who helped to find someone who had access to a computer, and they did the forms online.

Only by talking honestly about his poor prognosis did Kenny come to the realisation that things needed putting into place. As we talked, it became clear that Kenny thought he had many years ahead to live. I gently explained that this might be overly optimistic: it wouldn't surprise me that his next birthday could well be his last. After the shock of hearing this, Kenny took some time to think and it felt like we were both now aware of the seriousness of his illness. He began to appreciate how short the time ahead might be, and though he was deeply troubled by this, he was keen to get more in control of his life again. It took weeks of negotiation, yet it was well worth it: we developed a safer plan and Kenny now feels that the situation is more bearable.

'There are days,' he tells me, 'when I don't feel too bad and have a good one. I'm thinking of going down the pub at the weekend. There are days when I'm just too tired and stay in bed. But at least I know why, so I'm not too worried.'

Going to the pub may not be your priority, but for Kenny it's been achievable and made life a little easier. He's given Lucy to Ian, who brings her round every day for a snack and a cuddle. And it's not just Kenny and Ian who are now aware that time is short; so are my team at the surgery. If Kenny calls, we know to respond quickly. We've also alerted the Out-of-Hours services to Kenny's situation, as well as the local ambulance headquarters. If there's a problem and he calls for help, then the people who arrive to assist should know Kenny's case and his wishes. This is called 'Advance Care Planning', which we'll look at in detail in a few pages. The idea is to make decisions early on and let people around you and those involved in your health care know what those decisions are. I appreciate that your situation is different from Kenny's, and you may well not be at a similar point right now, but it's worth considering these issues. We'll return to delve deeper into the legal aspects of planning in Chapter 10.

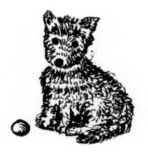

EXAMPLE 2

I met Janey at the hospice. She was 29, and diagnosed with ovarian cancer three years ago. It had spread and her situation was deteriorating. She was a single mum with a six-year-old daughter, Alice. Alice was everything to Janey. She wanted as much time as possible to spend with Alice.

This was so hard. I knew there was not much time ahead for Janey: I could tell from the scan reports that showed widespread disease, from her rapid weight loss, her increasing fatigue, and from the fact she was having increasing difficulty caring for Alice on her own.

Our discussion was lengthy and clearly distressing.

'Janey, it feels like things are changing. Have you noticed that?'

'What do you mean?'

'Well, since I saw you you've lost some more weight. You seem to me to be more tired.'

'Yes. Yes, I am more tired. It's so worrying.'

'Which part is so worrying?'

'I'M GOING TO DIE!' she shouted this at me. And that's OK. These questions can seem awkward and awful no matter how kindly we ask them. I let some time pass and I started again.

'Can you tell me what is important for you now?'

'I want to be able to look after Alice.'

'What's stopping you doing that?'

'I'm so tired now. And I feel sick a lot.'

'If we could improve your tiredness a little and reduce your sickness would that be enough?'

'No.' Long pause. *'I need someone to help me at home. And I need someone to look after her when I'm gone.'*

Although this conversation was very distressing, we had a glimmer of a way forward. Janey started on anti-sickness medication along with a low dose of a steroid called Dexamethasone for her fatigue. Her symptoms improved a little, but, disappointingly, not dramatically. What really helped was getting one of Janey's family to come and help with Alice. Her niece, 15, moved in, and though she was young she was able to help Alice to get up in the morning, give her breakfast, walk her to school and then go to school herself. She then picked up Alice from after-school club and brought her home. Janey had rested most of the day and felt able then to take over. This small intervention did more than any tablet, and the next time I met Janey she was much calmer. We were able to talk through options as to who might look after Alice. Janey never asked me how much time was ahead. I think she was too scared of the answer. Instead we worked together on what mattered most to her, and the end result was as good as it could have been in this tragic scenario.

2.2ii Planning options – your hopes and dreams for the time you have left

Meanwhile, back to you. As well as being individual in terms of our ability to tolerate treatment, **we're all different in terms of our desires, wishes and dreams. What matters to me won't be the same as what matters to you.** I can't say exactly how I'll feel in the future, but I'm pretty certain that for me, having more time ahead will be

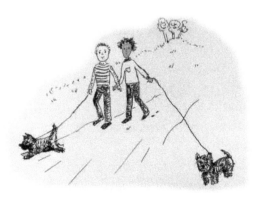

less important than the ability to be at home, feeling as well as I can, with my loved ones, doing the things I like doing.

What about for you? And remember, this isn't a bucket list of things to tick off like in a Hollywood movie. It's not about flying to the moon or climbing Everest or winning a Nobel Prize: **it's an assurance that you can do the things you treasure and be with the people you love in as much comfort and with as much presence as you can.**

TIP: Ask yourself: if I have six months or even six weeks left to live, what is most important for me?

OPTION 1: Written Notes

It can be helpful to write down the things *you do and don't want to happen in your future care.* There isn't a legal obligation to make these things happen, but it gives guidance to those around you who can try to make sure they do. Here are some desires I have seen written down:

- If anything happens to me I want my cat with me at all times.
- I would like to go France one more time.
- I don't want to go back to hospital.
- I want to see my granddaughter Emily as soon as possible.
- I want to make up with next door, as we fell out over the fence.
- I like to sleep with three pillows, including the one I made myself.
- I have a strong Jewish faith and I want my rabbi to help arrange my funeral.
- I want to be scattered on the lake where we went boating last summer.
- Please make sure no one touches my crucifix, it's important to me that I have it with me at all times.
- I have paid for my burial plot, and the details are in my filing cabinet top drawer
- I would like to die outdoors so I can hear the birds singing.

41

You'll find space to jot down a few of your dreams, wishes and desires at the end of this chapter. Alternatively, you might prefer to use an NHS resource[6] to create an Advance Care Plan or Statement.

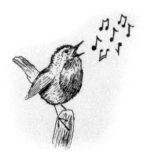

OPTION 2: An Advance Care Plan or Statement

TIP: An Advance Care Plan is a written statement that documents your health situation alongside your wishes and hopes for your future care. It's not the same as an Advance Decision to Refuse Treatment (ADRT). This used to be called a Living Will, and we will look at it in more detail in Chapter 10. But it's a good place to keep an ADRT if you have one.

You can formalise your **wishes** for your care in a written document called an Advance Care Plan. You can write this plan with support from relatives, carers, health or social care professionals and it can cover any aspect of your future health or social care. **Whilst the focus is on what is important to you, it helps to include your diagnosis, your next-of-kin details, letters from hospital and your current medication.** It differs from a Living Will or Advance Decision to Refuse Treatment, which is a legally binding document stating your **decisions** around refusing specific medical interventions, and we will look more into this in Chapter 11. To be clear, the difference between these documents is the difference between documenting your **wishes** and your legally formed **decisions**. The Dying Matters website (www.dyingmatters.org) is a good resource if you would like further clarification.

TIP: Be wary of your loved ones wanting what they feel is best for you and of strong opinions within your family, and be mindful of your wanting to satisfy others rather than yourself.

Your Advance Care Plan could include all the aspirations listed above, as well as:

- How you want any religious or spiritual beliefs you hold to be reflected in your care.
- Where you would like to be cared for as you become frailer – it could be home, hospital, a care home, or hospice.
- How you like to do things – for example, if you prefer a shower instead of a bath, or like to sleep with the light on.
- Concerns about practical issues – for example, who will look after your cat or dog if you become ill.

TIP: Ideally sign and date your Advance Care Plan, then it's clear that it's yours. You can change your mind at any time by changing the documentation, and then signing and dating the changes.

An Advance Care Plan is not legally binding, but it should be taken into account by those responsible for your care.

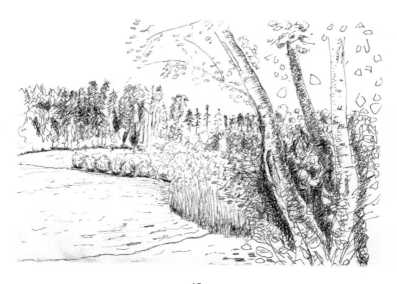

2.3 A quick recap

In summary, **it's hard to predict the future.** Clinicians are not soothsayers or palm readers. Doctors have to rely on experiences we have had, and also the variations that prove the exceptions to the rule.

TIP: Rather than thinking about how much time lies ahead, it can be more helpful to focus on what matters most to you.

Making your wishes known with some Advance Care Planning, whilst you are well and have the ability to communicate, can help those around you support you.

Which brings us neatly to the next chapter – reaching out to our loved ones, our medical teams, our support network – and finding help. That way, we can make what's important to us happen.

For your own notes:

....

....

....

....

....

....

....

....

....

II. BEING CARED FOR

3. REACHING OUT FOR HELP FROM YOUR FAMILY AND FRIENDS

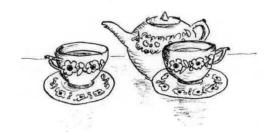

'When my cancer returned for the second time, I knew it was bad news, and that was all I could deal with. I didn't want to know the prognosis, and I didn't want to talk to anyone about it. Every time I did, I'd get so upset, I'd start crying, and it just made things worse.' **Paul, 44**

'I can talk to Ken. We've been together 50 years and he is my best friend. We've been planning my funeral together as I'm good at organising and I know he'll struggle with it otherwise. I've found it surprisingly cathartic.' **Dorothy 83**

'What's the point in talking? It's not going to change anything, is it?' **Danny, 32**

Our thoughts and feelings around illness are as individual as we are, and so is the way we communicate about them. Some of us gladly talk to our friends and family members in order that everyone is up to speed on the situation, others prefer to confide in the one person who is close to us. There are those who find it easier to chat to strangers, whilst some prefer to put their trust in health professionals and only to be open with them.

Moreover, it's not just a question of who we talk to, it's also about how much we decide to tell. Some people seem to find it easy to talk about what's going on, for others it's almost impossible. As we discussed in the previous chapter, some people want to be told everything clearly and plainly, and are able to be just as frank with those around them. For others, privacy is key. Perhaps this stems from fear of causing pain and upset, perhaps from a fear dying. Or maybe it's caused by a desire to hold onto one's dignity, or worries such as work finding out. Often it's a combination of several of these things.

Whichever way you live with your illness, **the easiest way forward is to share with those around you the key things that are important to you,** whether they are simple and obvious, or wild and extreme.

'My therapist has been amazing. She's spent so much time with me and the girls that I feel she's family now. My girls are so young, and it's so hard to explain what's happening. She's really helped me find my way.' **Karin, 51**

3.1 Support from your family and friends

For most of us it's important to spend as much time as possible in our own homes, using a support network to help make that happen. We'll return to the practicalities of care at home in Chapter 5, but here we'll look at communicating with those immediately around you, in the hope we can make it easier for all involved.

3.1i Communicating with your loved ones

TIP: Take some time to consider how open you want to be.

- If you want privacy, do say so. Some people prefer to cope by *not* talking about their illness at all. Nobody wants to force you to talk through issues you'd rather avoid, and if you're not comfortable doing so, it's OK to tell people this.
- Beware of a 'conspiracy of silence', where everyone skirts around the plain truth, trying not to talk about it. This tends to make matters even more distressing.
- Think about who you would like to talk to. This may be obvious when you're with your partner, but less so if you are living alone. You still may have a number of people around wanting to help, but who might be best placed, say, to come to appointments? Someone else might be in a better position to mow the lawn or do the laundry.

TIP: You can document your wishes around communication and information in your Advance Care Statement (see previous chapter), and these wishes can also be incorporated into your medical record.

A NOTE ABOUT BOUNDARIES

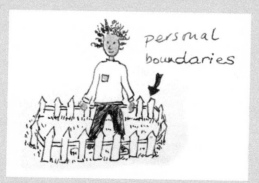

Psychologically, the borders or limits we set for ourselves in relation to others vary from one individual to another: what's OK for me physically, emotionally, socially or sexually may not be OK for you. Although we're all different, it's possible to generalise: **people with healthy boundaries make good choices about who they trust and how much they trust them; people with unhealthy boundaries can be vulnerable to others taking advantage of them**. If you're the sort of person who finds it hard to assert your needs around other people, or who often says 'yes' because it's easier, or who tends to tell people what they want to hear rather than speaking the truth, chances are your boundaries may be on the weaker side. Having weaker boundaries is not wrong, but it's just worth reminding yourself that *you* are the most important person here. It's all too easy to end up taking care of others, and in the process this might mean you forget to look after yourself.

3.1ii Asking for help

Sarah has pointed out that it's not always easy to ask for help. Some of us find it easy to lean on others, but often there's a little voice that stops us, saying we 'should' manage on our own.

'Today, I went to a social gathering outside in a garden with a lovely lunch buffet. In the past it wouldn't have been a problem for me, but since my stroke I'm not that steady on my feet, and it's affected my eyesight, so I find it hard to gauge distances, and how flat or sloping the ground is. My daughter had taken me, but she was chatting to the host, and suddenly acquiring food at a buffet seemed an impossible task. I didn't want to bother her; they're old friends and hadn't seen each other in a while.

'There were plenty of offers of help, but I spent most of the lunch trying to do things on my own. Why? Partly it was the practicality: I'm a fussy eater so "Can I get you a plate of food" wasn't going to work for me. Partly it was fear of inconveniencing someone: I don't want to inflict myself on them. It was also a lack of trust.

'But when my daughter saw me struggling to get back to my seat with a plate, she said "Oh mum! Why didn't you call me?" and later, I realised that it's a case of wanting to do it all myself, of still wanting to be seen as independent and capable. My brain is telling me that I should be able to do it all by myself. There are two flaws I can see in that thinking. Firstly, accepting help doesn't necessarily mean that I can't do a thing. It's just easier with someone alongside me. And secondly, why "should" I be able to do everything? How absurd. I don't have to be able to juggle my symptoms, a plate, and those things you use to serve up salad. It doesn't make me a failure as a human, just a normal person who is recovering from a stroke!

'My pride was getting in the way and making life that little bit more difficult. As with a lunch buffet, so with the bigger things in life. There are days where I can get through mostly by myself, but a chat with a friend or a hug makes it that much easier. And there are times when I can't get through the day without help from others, and that's alright too.' **Elsa, 69**

'What Elsa is describing is common, but it's also important to differentiate between pride and dignity,' says Sarah. 'When we're at our most vulnerable, it's important for people to retain their identity – and this is true at the end of life, too. My stepfather, Adrian, did not want my mum, or me, helping him to go the loo. He had a stoma[7] and he dealt with it on his own for over two years, but when he got to the point that he was too weak to manage it, that was when he said he'd like to get assistance from outside, rather than have us do it, and we organised for a professional carer to visit twice a day. We had to pay for it, but he didn't have long left by this point, and it mattered a lot to him that he could still be the man he wanted to be. With hindsight, it was good for us, too. It meant we could do the "nice" things, and I have a poignant memory of rubbing soothing ointment into his feet, which were very dry. He was happy for me to do that, but dealing with his bowels was off limits.'

3.2i Friends and neighbours

Not everyone has someone nearby, or gets on with their family. It may be important to include someone outside of your family circle to help negotiate the ways forward. In any event, friends can often give you things your close family can't.

'When Pete told me his cancer had returned and there was nothing they could do, initially I wasn't sure what to say. I felt a bit awkward to be honest. But he said it was good that I was just there to listen and hang out, having a bit of a laugh. I do have a bit of a dark sense of humour and I guess I've found the perfect avenue for it. Sometimes we just watch the football or do the Soduko together in the paper, sometimes we don't do anything much at all, but he said just having me there was what mattered.' **Leon, 59**

3.3 Care for those who are caring for you

'When I was struggling with high levels of anxiety, one bit of advice really stuck with me. It's that familiar message from the flight attendant at the start of the flight. "In the event of an emergency, please put on your oxygen mask before assisting others." If you're caring for someone else it's so easy to forget this. But it's crucial: you need to take care of yourself in order to be effective in supporting someone else – because without an oxygen mask on yourself, you're no good to anyone.' **Sarah**

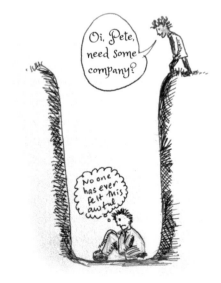

If you are a carer, is there someone to look after you? Carers often struggle and also need support.

Signs that you might be struggling include:

- Fatigue
- Poor sleep
- Falls
- Feeling low
- Poor attention
- Anger and frustration

If you're beginning to feel like this, Sarah has some basic advice:

TIPS FOR RELATIVES AND FRIENDS:

- **Do something physical** – self-care can quickly turn into self-neglect when we lose focus of our physical bodies and what we need. Build in time to exercise, even if it's just a short walk, and try to make sure you're getting enough sleep.
- **Talk to your own friends and other family members to let off steam** – sometimes those you are caring for are difficult to be around. Not all, by any means, but if this true for you, it's OK to say 'my mum is driving me mad!' and it's better you share your frustration with others than get angry with the person you are caring for.
- **Block out time for yourself –** if you're caring for someone who is very, very sick you may well want to be with them as much as you can. But sometimes the process of dying is gradual. Such was the case with my father, for instance, who was diagnosed with Alzheimer's, a life-limiting illness, over a decade before he died. In this sort of situation it can be hard to find time for yourself, and you may feel guilty about it, but it's vital if you are to take care of your own mental health over the longer term. If you're feeling worn

out, please ask a friend or other family member to take over the care for a bit to allow you to recuperate. There are often local services specifically aimed at supporting family member(s) who are spending a lot of their lives caring. Having a break can be achieved through respite care or by having a temporary agency help to fill in.

- If you are a carer, **you may also worry about what might happen if you become unwell.** For example, if you look after someone with dementia, and become ill yourself, who will look after them? Often family members will step in, but there is also help via Social Services. **In an emergency, there is usually a team (in our area this is called the Intermediate Care Team) who can assess a patient's needs urgently, putting care swiftly into place either at home or in a care home as needed.** They can be accessed via your GP, district nurse, Macmillan Nurse or Social Services directly.

There is more information at Carers UK: 020 7378 4999 www.carersuk.org. You'll find some more useful tips on giving support at mariecurie.org.uk[8] and on many of the charity websites listed at the end of the book.

4. HELP FROM YOUR HEALTHCARE TEAMS

'I didn't know what a GP really did, but over the weeks she's really helped me, not just with how I feel physically, but by listening too. She's made me feel safe.' **Kandy, 24**

As I look at the long list of health experts, websites and support groups we've pulled together in this book, it strikes me how many people are willing to help. Perhaps they've made a career out of helping others, or their passion springs from experience with friends or family members, or from faith, or perhaps it's the result of being patients themselves. There is a lot of support out there so do take advantage of it – it's for you.

4.1i Your GP and the Primary Care Team

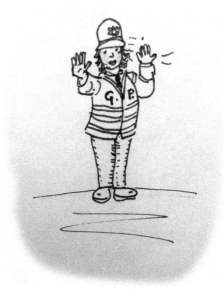

Not only do we GPs actively support and treat patients with symptoms as they arise, but we can also direct patients to the large variety of useful people and places that can also help. Think of your GP as also being like a traffic police officer, say, directing you to where you need to go. If you'd like to talk to someone about your illness, I suggest you make your GP your first port of call. Book an appointment with the doctor at your practice whom you feel most comfortable with and trust.

TIP: Before you see your doctor, write a list of your concerns. As mentioned earlier, it's a good idea to bring someone with you, who can support and prompt you.

> *'I try to go to my mother's health appointments with her, and if for some reason I can't, then I arrange for someone else to accompany her. Often there are things I remember to ask or say that Mum has forgotten, but sometimes it's the other way round. Last week at the dentist mum said, "You've forgotten to tell her I'm on Warfarin," and I said, "So I have," and explained she's on a dose of 5.5mg, and Mum interrupted to say, "No, that was last week. Now I'm on 6.5!"'* **Sarah**

Not everyone has a relative locally, so this isn't always possible. **If you're alone and are concerned you might forget your GP's advice, ask them to explain or write the key points down.** They may recommend speaking to a specialist nurse or your hospital consultant, or they might suggest things you hadn't thought of, such as a local counselling service.

TIPS FOR DEALING WITH YOUR GP:

- **If the receptionist isn't being helpful, ask for a phone consultation so you can talk directly to your GP.**
- If you're still having issues with getting support from your GP, which is mercifully rare, then **consider attending Out-of-Hours GP services if symptoms need addressing urgently**.
- You can think about changing GP if you aren't happy with them. It's easy to do and won't interfere with your care. Ask around for recommendations, then go into the surgery you want to change to, with your repeat prescription, proof of your address, photo identification and sign up. It's also an idea to get internet access. You can then access your record online in order to book appointments or order repeat

medication. There's even an app to use on your phone to do the same! Which site and app will depend on which software system your practice uses. The common ones are:

- EMIS patient.emisaccess.co.uk/Account/Login
- VISION myvisiononline.co.uk/vpp/
- SYSTMONE tpp-uk.com/products/systmonline

4.2 Nurses – who's who?

Alongside your GP, there are a large number of groups willing to help and support you. For almost every disease type there is a supportive clinical network.

1. At a local level this is your GP surgery and District Nurse team.
2. At a broader Primary Care level, depending on your diagnosis, this might be your community Clinical Nurse Specialist (CNS), such as the Macmillan, Respiratory, and Heart Failure nurses.
3. At the hospital, a similar set of Clinical Nurse Specialists (CNSs) operate, and they are there to provide continuity and support for patients passing though their department.

Let's have a look at these in more detail.

- **District Nurses (DNs).** Based in the community, DNs provide the backbone of home support for those with terminal illnesses. Their role is to provide interventions, such as wound dressing and medication injections, and also to help refer you on to other agencies such as the Occupational Therapist or Social Worker. They can make up to three or four visits a day in times of crisis, but they are not there to provide 24-hour cover. They will visit from two to three times a day if need be, with shifts providing night-time visits. But more rural areas don't benefit from this service, and some inner city areas don't fund 24-hour nursing, so it can be hit and miss. They can help organise night sits, if available, from services such as Marie Curie nurses: 0800 0902309 mariecurie.org.uk/help/nursing-services or the local Hospice at Home team if available in your are nahh.org.uk/about-hospice-care/what-is-hospice-at-home.

- **Palliative Care (Macmillan) Clinical Nurse Specialist (CNS).** There are misconceptions around what a palliative care Macmillan nurse does. To clarify, they explore your history with you, take a look at your symptoms and medication, note your social setting and finances, and get an idea as to what your prognosis might be. They then make a plan with you of what support is needed, and who may help to provide that support. There is an expectation that palliative care Macmillan nurses will be at your bedside like Florence Nightingale, at all hours of the day and night. But that sort of hands-on care usually comes from family members with support from a combination of District Nursing and carer staff, who are less specialised but highly skilled. Macmillan nurses tend to work 9-5, and use their expertise to advise your GP and District Nurses about your care. They talk to you about whatever physical and emotional symptoms you have, assess what medication may help you, and direct you to services such as counselling, hospice day care, and social services. Though personal experiences can vary, they usually

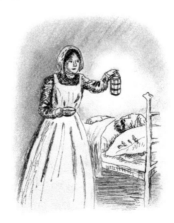

provide a fantastic service, partly through their expertise and kindness, and partly by making sure everyone is working together for your good.

'I've found that Sheila, my Macmillan Nurse, has more time to talk through my day-to-day concerns than my consultant. My consultant gave me the diagnosis, she helps me with my physical symptoms and the bigger picture.' **Ben**

- **Other Specialist Nurses**. These include Heart Failure, COPD or Respiratory, Parkinson's, Diabetes CNSs, and Admiralty Nurses for dementia. Again, rather than just speaking to the doctor, CNSs are skilled in helping you solve a problem, such as explaining your medication regimen, prescribing medication themselves, and addressing practical issues such as oxygen home delivery.

4.3 Your Consultant and the Hospital Team

This is the hospital doctor with the expertise around your condition. They will explain the treatment schedule. This may include surgery, medication, radiotherapy, chemotherapy, or any combination of these. If your clinic is busy, you may see one of the training team. Let's have a look at the badges the training doctors wear and what they mean:

- A Registrar (Specialist Trainee ST3-6) is training to be a consultant in that specialty.
- A Core Trainee (CT1-2), is on a career path to becoming a Registrar.
- A GP trainee (ST1-3) gains training experience by working in a hospital.
- A Foundation Year doctor (FY1-2) is the most junior doctor, a year or two out of qualifying, who works in outpatient clinics and on the wards to gain experience.

The more junior the doctor, the more likely that they will need to speak to the consultant to make sure that their decision-making is correct. Ideally this is a safe system, with consultant back up for advice.

- Each consultant has a secretary. They usually work 8.30am – 4pm, and most are part-time. Find out when the secretary works, as they are often a key contact to help with, for example, changing appointments, re-organising follow-up, or simply someone to pass your thanks on to if things have gone well.

'Recently, I had to move my appointment and Robin, my consultant's secretary was a godsend.' **Sonia, 57**

TIP: Before you get too embroiled in finding out everything about your illness from a specialist consultant, again, check in with yourself: What do I need to know? What do I want to know? What do I feel comfortable knowing?

- **Hospital Macmillan Nurse (CNS)**. Hospital Macmillan nurses work with patients with cancer. They usually have a specialism, such as lung cancer or breast cancer and help to navigate you through your cancer treatment and subsequent follow up. They should be able to answer questions as diverse as 'What kind of chemotherapy will I get?' and 'Will I feel sick?' to 'What happens if I miss a treatment or don't feel well enough?' Ask away! If they don't know, they will find someone who does. They are also good at finding out what's gone wrong if an expected scan hasn't been booked or a result seems to be a long time coming. Once your treatment is finished, the CNS can then transfer your care onto the Palliative Care team CNS, if appropriate, who will provide ongoing support when you are at home. We'll touch more on Palliative Care in a few pages.
- **Other Hospital Clinical Nurse Specialists (CNS)** – as with the community, hospitals also have specialist nursing

services. Sometimes they work in both the community and the hospital. Like the Macmillan team, they are specialised in specific disease areas, and can provide treatment and sign-posting support to other services such as social care.

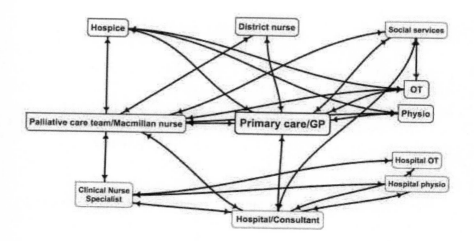

Once you find support, you might be pleasantly surprised by how much is out there. But a familiar story I hear is that a person gets a diagnosis and then feels isolated and abandoned because they are not yet within the system that I've outlined above. Let's have a look at Karen's story, then at Pete's better experience.

EXAMPLE 1

Karen was diagnosed with breast cancer on Friday afternoon at the hospital. She hadn't been expecting a bad diagnosis, so had gone to the appointment on her own. She came home, devastated, and couldn't remember any of the details that had been explained to her in the clinic. She'd also misplaced the leaflets she'd been given. Her family were just as upset, and didn't know what was happening or how to find help. They called Out of Hours, who advised speaking to their GP on Monday. But this was two days away. On Monday they contacted the GP, but the surgery had no further information as they hadn't heard from the hospital. They advised Karen to contact the

Breast Care Nurse at the local hospital, and gave her the number. The Nurse was able to deal with Karen's concerns and organised for her to come back to clinic to go through the diagnosis again, this time with a member of her family present. She also gave Karen the number for Macmillan Cancer Care to get more information on finances.

EXAMPLE 2

Pete went to the respiratory clinic with his wife Joan. The consultant told him he had pulmonary fibrosis, and they were going to start him on a new treatment. Pete's dad had died of a lung condition, so he started remembering that, and wasn't paying attention to what the doctor said. Joan asked a few questions, but they came out feeling at a loss. Chris, the respiratory CNS, saw them looking bewildered and asked if they were OK.

'Not really,' said Pete. 'I keep thinking how my dad died and it was awful.'

Chris took them into a side-room. 'What happened to your dad?' she asked.

'He had lung cancer. Coughed and spluttered, shouting and screaming till he died,' said Pete.

'I'm really sorry to hear that. And it isn't my experience with patients who have lung cancer these days. It's worth noting, Pete, that what you have is a different disease. I don't see any of that happening to you.'

They talked through Pete's condition, what medication they were thinking of trying, and what would happen next.

Joan asked, 'If he gets sicker can he stay at home or will he have to be here on oxygen?'

'We'll continue to monitor Pete's condition, and as things change then home adaptations could be put into place, including portable oxygen' said Chris.

She wrote down her number and the consultant's secretary's number, and then arranged a follow-up appointment.

By the time Pete and Joan came to see me at the GP surgery, I'd had a letter from the hospital explaining the diagnosis, the plan of action, and I could talk it through with them both. We had a clear starting point.

For HOSPITAL SUPPORT, ask for the name and phone numbers of your consultant, their secretary and the nurse specialist. You will also need the Chemotherapy Hotline number if you are undergoing treatment.

For HOME SUPPORT, get the District Nurse's number – both day and night ones as they tend to be different. Have your GP Out-of-Hours number to hand. There is often also 24-hour information from your local hospice helpline number. Write the numbers down (you could jot them below) or put them on your phone and keep them safe. Then you have them altogether in advance, should you need help at any time.

Support line phone numbers:

....

....

....

....

....

....

TIP: If you feel you haven't got the information you need, or aren't clear about what's happening, then speak to the receptionist or your Clinical Nurse Specialist before you leave the clinic. The CNS is often the person best placed to understand where you are on your journey and how to fix an issue.

4.3i Transport to and from hospital

Unfortunately, in these increasingly impoverished times in terms of NHS funding, patients are expected to get themselves to and from appointments, or to get family or friends to take them. It's really frustrating, especially if you have to go often for a course of treatment, which may be the case if you are having radiotherapy (see Chapter 9), for instance.

TIP: There is some recompense available from the NHS[9] according to which benefits you receive. Full details are on their website, as well as information on the forms you will need, including HC1 application form, as well as the HC2 and HC3[10] certificates.

'I couldn't afford the taxi there. The Macmillan nurse phoned me, and she managed to get my chemo moved to my local hospital. I didn't know they did it there.' **Arthur 88 – lymphoma**

Another option is the patient transport service (PTS). This is a local ambulance service that can take you to and from appointments if you are frail and unable to get to hospital yourself. If you need help, do call them to see if you are eligible – each area has different criteria as to what you need to qualify. But be warned that they will be taking several people so the journey is bound to be longer, and your wait will be too. The PTS ambulance will often pick you up at around 8am, and deliver you home any time after 6pm, along with other patients who live near you. This can be exhausting, and unfortunately I have seen it affect the desire of some of my patients to want to return to hospital. Experiences vary, and if you have a good service locally that is great. The plus side is that you will be with people who may be going through similar experiences and it can be helpful to exchange news and views on your journey.

'I met John on the bus to chemo. He made me laugh, made the whole thing bearable.' **Aggy, 78 – melanoma**

TIP: If you don't have someone to take you, and aren't eligible for PTS, ask at your GP surgery if there are alternative ways you can get help with transportation. At our surgery there is a *Friends and Neighbours* group that provides car transport for a donation, if booked in advance. The Red Cross[11] can also sometimes help you to get to and from appointments.

4.4 Your Palliative Care Team

There's one more group of people who are around to help you: the Palliative Care Team. You may have heard the term but not know exactly what it means, so let's pause for a definition: *palliative care is the active holistic care of patients with advanced progressive illness. Management of pain and other symptoms and provision of psychological, social and spiritual support is paramount. The goal of palliative care is achievement of the best quality of life for patients and their families*[12].

Palliative Care emerged from the hospice movement begun by Cicely Saunders in 1967. She realised that patients weren't getting adequate care at the end of their lives. From her early work, hospices emerged throughout the UK to support people dying of cancer. Over time, this remit extended to include all people with life-limiting illness. The services offered by hospices broadened, supporting people earlier in their journey as well as in the last weeks of life. Palliative Care Teams are also based in hospitals and within the community.

Palliative Care takes a 'holistic' approach, which means that it considers the whole person – body, mind, spirit and emotions – in the quest for optimal health and wellness. The Palliative Care Team aims to provide something broader than clinical care. The team consists of Palliative Medicine Consultants, Clinical Nurse Specialists (often titled Macmillan Nurses), Hospice Nurses, social workers, psychologists, physio- and occupational therapists; there is spiritual care from chaplaincy, and there is a variety of holistic therapists who focus on therapies such as art, music, drama and relaxation. There are many volunteers involved as well, giving their time to hospice services, driving patients to and from appointments, and generally helping out.

4.4i Allied healthcare professionals

As well as at the hospice, you can access support within the community. Those involved in your palliative care can include:

- **A Physiotherapist** – usually accessed via your GP or hospital consultant. They can help with a variety of physical activities from exercises to strengthen muscles to hydrotherapy for stiffened limbs.
- **An Occupational Therapist** – again accessed via your doctor, CNS, or via Social Services. They can help by assessing mobility and ensuring that your home is as safe as it can be. They look at the risk of falling and can arrange for mobility aids such as handrails, zimmer frames and hand grabs for your bath. We'll talk more about this in Chapter 4.
- **A Dietician** – if you are struggling to get adequate nutrition then a dietician can help. They assess your calorie intake, the issues you have around eating such as swallowing, and can advise your doctor to prescribe nutritional supplements. This is particularly the case if you are receiving nutrition via a tube rather than by eating.
- **A Translator** – if English isn't your first language, an interpreter can be organised in advance for your consultation. Doctors try not to use family members to translate as this can be upsetting or cause misunderstandings. Try to let the clinic know in advance of the language that you need translating.
- **A Counsellor or Therapist** – it is common to struggle coping with a life-limiting illness, and we'll come on to talk more about looking after your mental health in Chapter 7. Access to counselling is usually from your GP, but you may find that the hospital team has specific support. This is more likely for conditions such as cancer and motor neurone disease (MND). Again, the CNS should be able to tell you about any counselling that is available through their team.

4.5 Hospices

'I dreaded the word "Hospice". But when I got there everyone was so nice. They really listened. I look forward to going on a Tuesday. I get lunch, a massage, and then there's the relaxation session where everything seems to stop for a while.' **Anna, 88**

Your local hospice is a palliative care service, run as a charity, using funds raised by the local community with a smaller portion from your local health authority. The services hospices offer vary, but can include:

- **Day hospice care.** Patients usually attend once a week for holistic support: this means support for the whole body and mind, which comes from the nursing, physiotherapy, chaplaincy, counselling, alternative therapy team, and whoever else is around to help. There is also the benefit of spending time with other people who are also living with serious illness. They have experiences, knowledge and their worries to share, as will you. This is a great opportunity to get support. Inpatient doctors can be called in to give medical support, but on the whole these are nurse-led days, focusing on support over weeks. Courses run can include *Living with Breathlessness, Living with Advanced Illness,* and even courses for carers such as *Living With Someone With Dementia.*
- **Inpatients.** Admissions to the ward can be for better control of symptoms, with the aim of discharge home once this is done. It can also be a place to die, for the last days of life. For some patients they have spent some time at the day hospice and feel like they would like to end their days there. For a few patients, their symptoms are complex leading to difficulties controlling them at home: hospice can provide the 24-hour medical and nursing expertise to help manage them. Times of admission vary from hospice to hospice, but they usually take patients in the mornings from Monday to Friday. Out of Hours admissions are done rarely, as it's not

the best way to deal with issues arising when the full hospice team aren't present. The team are better placed to help in advance – so call during the day if difficulties are creeping in. The usual length of stay is up to two weeks, but this is negotiated on an individual basis according to need. A decision will be made as to whether continuing at the hospice is the right thing to do or whether, after stabilisation, future care can be undertaken at home, or at a residential or nursing home.

- **Outpatients.** Here you can be seen by the Palliative Care Consultant or one of their team for more detailed assessment and management of your situation and symptoms.

- **Lymphoedema clinic.** Some cancers are associated with swelling caused by leakage of fluid from the blood vessels into the surrounding tissue. This is known as lymphoedema. Specialist lymphoedema nurses can offer massage and advice around compression stockings and skin care to minimise the discomfort this causes.

- **Alternative therapies.** These can include aromatherapy, massage, relaxation, breathing exercises, reflexology, acupuncture – a wide array of kind and calming therapies to make you feel better. The services available locally will vary. Some hospices have hydrotherapy pools, some have calm, darkened relaxation rooms. Ask what's available at yours. What would you like? What might help you to feel a little easier today?

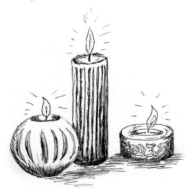

WHAT'S THE DIFFERENCE BETWEEN A HOSPICE, A CARE HOME AND A NURSING HOME?

- Care homes are split into two types. Firstly, there are residential homes, for those who need 24-hour support but no nursing input.
- Secondly, there are nursing homes, for those with complex needs who require extra nursing input. This can include administration of medication via PEG tubes, helping to manage oxygen masks, and assistance for those who cannot care for themselves physically, such as after a stroke.
- Hospices differ by providing an intensive medical environment that aims to get symptoms controlled with an aim to discharge, if the patient is not within the last days of life, to home or to a care home.

All three settings offer care for the last days of life, but the hospice stay is usually temporary. In residential homes, District Nurses will attend to provide additional nursing needs as required.

4.6 Getting help and support from charities

Numerous charities exist dedicated to raising awareness about illness and providing support for those suffering from them. You'll find a full, if not exhaustive, list at the end of this book on page 197 – if you flip to have a quick look, you can see that there are *lots* of charities out there. It's worth taking the time to find the one most suitable for you. If you are in doubt, your GP or Clinical Nurse Specialist should be able to point you to the most appropriate charity for your condition. The people who work there want to help you, and you will find support provided by telephone, internet, or in some cases by direct contact with their workers.

TIP: Remember, you don't have to be the patient to contact the charity. Someone can do this on your behalf to start the ball rolling. Your loved one can also call for advice. PLEASE DON'T BE AFRAID OF CALLING. These support groups are there for you.

'I felt so alone. I went to the website and had a moan in one of the chatrooms. It felt good talking to someone else who had my illness.'
Chrissy, 22

'I don't know why I waited, but I didn't call them for a month. Daft really, 'cos they were lovely on the phone and really got where I was coming from.' **Rhys, 67**

There is also good practical support available from the following national agencies:

- **Age UK:** 0800 169 2081, ageuk.org.uk
  This is the charity for older age. There will be a branch near you or, if you live more remotely, they have support on the phone.
- **Citizens Advice:** 0345 404 0506, citizensadvice.org.uk
  Citizens Advice can help with support around the law and social care.
- **The Red Cross:** 0344 871 1111, redcross.org.uk
  We often think that The Red Cross provide support abroad, but they also provide help close to home. Their help is often needed at times of crisis.

You will also find that information from non-charity sources is available on the internet – but be careful! Check that the site you're visiting is giving you reliable information. They can be skewed in one direction based on an overly positive or negative experience. Chat rooms, where people with the same illness can discuss their experiences, can vary in quality and safety. **Make sure you're safe online, please, dear reader**. If you come across something that is causing you alarm, try not to panic, though sometimes that can be easier said than done. **Remember there is often no one to verify stories online, and what you are reading may not be true!** If you pick up information you're unsure of please check with your medical team.

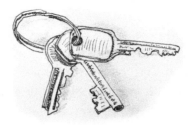

4.7 Getting help in an emergency

If you get unexpected worsening of your symptoms, feel feverish and unwell, are vomiting, or having difficulty breathing then you are likely to need medical help.

> **111 is the common Out Of Hours GP service. Check with your surgery to see if they use this number or if they have their own arrangements. Do this before you need them! 999 is the emergency number in the UK. The person answering calls will ask which service you need – choose *ambulance*. A crew will come to where you are and assess if you need admission to hospital.**

We can get other illnesses on top of our pre-existing condition, from chest and urine infections to blood clots and strokes, which can create a flare of crisis within your already troubling time of crisis. There is also the possibility of having more than one terminal illness. If your case is complex, then don't wait: please seek help quickly.

TIP: If you are receiving chemotherapy your local hospital will usually have given you a 'hotline' phone number for you to contact for advice. Make sure this is stored on your phone, or in a

place of visibility. If you develop a fever or feel unwell they are likely to direct you to your local A&E, especially if your temperature is above 38°C. Don't take paracetamol until you have spoken to the hotline for advice!!!

Chemotherapy can affect your immune system, making it more likely to get an infection. The raised temperature can be a sign that you have an infection that your suppressed immune system can't fight. Both oral and intravenous chemotherapy can cause these reactions. You are likely to need intravenous fluids and antibiotics in this situation.

TIP: Falls are common – if you can't get off the floor you will likely need help. Pendant alarms can be worn around the neck or on the wrist, and are available usually through Social Services. When pushed they alert services that you need help. Following a fall, a call to the ambulance service can also be appropriate as the crews are trained and skilled in helping people get up, getting back into bed, or assessing if they need admission to check for any broken bones.

My general advice on emergencies is don't wait. If you're worried, speak to someone sooner rather than later. Things can change quickly and are harder to remedy further down the line.

Some people hate going to hospital, others feel reassured by the 24-hour presence of nurses. If hospital is what you need, then it's likely that a specific treatment can't be given at home. If you are really adamant about not wanting to be admitted then you need to let people know. Decisions are often easier to make in advance whilst you are feeling stable and relatively well. Having said that, if you decide to change your mind that's fine too! It's *your* life, it's *your* body, and it's right and proper that you take charge of what's important to you.

5. HELP FOR YOU AT HOME FROM SOCIAL SERVICES

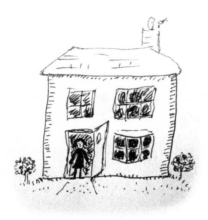

'Jeanie my carer comes by twice a day, and at first I was suspicious of a stranger coming into my house. But we get on brilliantly now. Bless her, she really lights up my day.' **Dolly, 98**

Where we live and who we live with greatly affects how we cope with illness. Living alone, living with our parents, living with children, living in the city or in the wild rural outback, these all colour our experience. On top of this our income matters hugely. Can we *afford* to be ill? In this chapter we'll look at Social Services, and the 'safety net' it offers in this time of crisis.

Larger families can have a mix of dynamics, some coping well and others coping poorly with sick relatives. I have patients who live alone who manage extremely well, happy with their own company and wishing to stay in their own houses, and sadly the exact opposite, with solitary patients struggling at home.

Access to where we live has an impact too – stairs that make wheelchair accessibility hard, lifts that don't work, roads that are too narrow for an ambulance – you get the picture. It's also important to recognise the difficulties of access to local services and hospitals, which may be miles away.

Given all these variables, it's worth thinking about who is around to help when you're not feeling up to it. Is their support enough? For some patients the easy answer is *'my family will sort it out'*. If it isn't straightforward, then referral to Social Services would be wise. Even if you are sure that you can manage OK, it's good to know there is extra help out there, as there may be days when you want to call on some expert assistance, especially if you are keen to stay at home for as long as possible, and **remember, most people with life-limiting illnesses are keen to remain in the place they know best.** I feel that way too, as I said in Chapter 1 – being in familiar surroundings, with my pets and loved ones close by.

If you have difficulty caring for yourself at home, Social Services can help you source assistance, from obtaining a pendant alarm for you to wear, to getting support from carers throughout the day. They can also assess you for benefits to which you may be entitled. The solution depends on a number of factors:

- What you would like
- What you can – and can't – afford
- What is available in your area

To start the process, you will need to contact your local Social Services department. They are located at your local council offices and are usually listed in your phone directory, if you have one, under Social Services. Alternatively, you can find your local office online using this link:

https://www.gov.uk/apply-needs-assessment-social-services

There is a specific team you will need called Adult Care Services.

5.1 Being assessed by Social Services

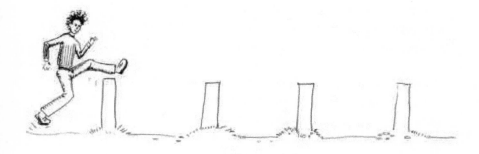

I'm going to keep this as simple as I can, but I'm afraid there are hurdles to get over. Social care can be really confusing even when you're thinking clearly; when you're reeling from a diagnosis it can be very hard. (In truth, I never quite understood how Social Services got separated from Health Care. If we're trying to consider the whole person, as those of us involved in palliative care aim to, it often seems so counterproductive. But here we are, with two systems that rarely speak to each other, both trying to care for the same person in their own ways.) Let me prepare you: there will be forms to fill in, bank statements to provide, phone calls and interviews at home. Sometimes it can feel like you are being interrogated about your personal and financial life. It seems unfair that these hurdles are put in your way when you're at your most fragile, but please try not to take it personally or feel that you've done anything wrong. The aim is to help you:

- Stay in your home as long as possible
- Access benefits you may be entitled to
- Get you access to carers who can help look after you
- Keep you as mobile and independent as possible

FACT: To access Social Services, you will need a referral.

This can be done by yourself or anyone you know, including your medical team, as long as they have your consent. It is usually done by phone. A family or friend may do it too. Sarah says she got in touch with Social Services on behalf of her mum, who is now registered for some support at home.

'When you have a needs assessment, it's a good idea to have a member of your family, a friend or a neighbour who knows you well with you. Even better if that person is someone who can be assertive yet patient and is good at admin! A tall order, I know, but they can help you feel safer and less overwhelmed, and also pick up on issues you may miss or forget to mention.' **Sarah**

5.1i Assessing your care needs

Once you've been referred, a social worker will pay a visit to make a 'Needs Assessment'[13]. This is an extensive assessment, looking at how you manage to look after yourself, from washing to feeding to shopping, to what kind of house you live in and who is around to help. **Together you will decide if you need to have carers come into your home** and how often they should visit. This is called a **'Package of Care'**. If care at home is decided upon, **then there needs to be a Financial Assessment** to look at how much you will contribute to your own care.

TIP: My advice is to get the Needs Assessment done early. You may not need any help now, but if there is a sudden change it's much easier to get input if the local Social Services team already knows your case.

5.1ii Assessing your finances

Money is a worry at the best of times, but when you're ill this can dominate matters. There is, however, some government provision to help. Many allowances are means-tested according to your income, but not all of them. Some money is available because you have a life-limiting illness, regardless of your income. Your Social Services team should help assess whether you can apply for Attendance Allowance, Personal Independence Payments (PIPs), and if there are grants available to help in certain circumstances. Some charities can help with finances too – it's worth looking on their websites, which are listed at the end of this book.

Broadly speaking, there is a threshold of savings that is allowable, currently £14,250, below which care is free. Between 14,250 and £23,250 in capital and savings, the council will contribute towards your care costs. Above that, you will have to fund all of your own social care. But this figure is changeable according to government policy, and the cap is due to alter significantly in 2020. Current advice is available from Age UK[14], where there is a calculator showing you what you may be entitled to. There is also more information on The Money Advice Service website[15].

FACT: There is a completely separate benefit called Attendance Allowance[16] *which is not means tested.* **If you are over 65 and are mentally or physically disabled and so need support, you should qualify. There are two levels: if you need help in the day you receive £55.65 a week; if you need help at night too, the amount is currently £83.10. Make sure you claim what you are entitled to – there is more information on benefits and the law in Chapter 10.**

TIP: **If, after your assessment, you think you're not getting what you are entitled to, then you can get help from Citizens Advice. Their details are in the web links section at the end of this book.**

5.1iii What sort of help might you get?

Here's an overview:

- **Even if you are entitled to free care, Social Services subcontract the work out which means that carers are**

usually provided by local private companies. If you are staying at home, the carer will visit from between 15 minutes to one hour depending on how much help you need. This can include help with dressing, help cooking, and prompting with medication. This means **the maximum carer time someone can receive free, via Social Services, is four hours a day. You may want to pay for extra care on top of this yourself.**

- If need increases, and four hours a day is inadequate to provide safe care at home, then a care home will provide more appropriate care. **Anytime something changes in your condition, a new 'needs assessment' needs to be arranged through the social worker to ensure you have the right package of care.**

- **Unfortunately a lot of people do not qualify for free care,** as the threshold in the UK is relatively low. This means you may be deemed to have resources to pay for your own care at home. This sounds as if it is bad news, and in many ways it is: using your savings to pay for healthcare is not what many wish for. The one advantage is that you can then organise care on your own terms. You can arrange a bespoke service – anything from one-off nursing care to having someone present 24-hours a day, if you can afford it. **If you go the self-funding route, you don't have to have a needs assessment, though it is important to keep your GP and Primary Care Team in the loop as to your arrangements.**

- **Care homes are also run privately and subcontract out to Social Services.** Funding for care homes has to meet strict criteria for Social Services to agree to it. If you have the means, you can pay for this care yourself. The average cost is around £850 a week, though this varies across the country. Advice on how to fund your care is available at the Age UK website. You can also call Age UK[17] on their helpline which is 0800 678 1174 for guidance.

'My dad and my stepmother, Dilys, were very keen that he should be able to stay in his own home, even though he had advanced Alzheimer's. The stress and upset of moving him to a care home would have been deeply distressing for them both at this stage in his life. He was very fortunate in that my stepmother was around to help and for many years she did most of the looking after of him, gradually increasing the amount of carer support she called upon. Although my father had sufficient savings so didn't qualify for free carer time via Social Services, Dilys felt it was much better to pay a private carer for a few hours a day than for him to be shifted somewhere else. It's hard to be away from the place you love when you are well, but with dementia, familiarity is often even more crucial. In his last weeks he had care for about six hours a day, but that was still more cost-effective than moving him. Every situation is different and what was right for my father may not be right for someone else, but in his circumstances, this seemed the wisest use of his funds and kindest way to look after him physically and mentally.' **Sarah**

'When Mum went into the care home we felt we had failed. But she blossomed. The company did her good, she ate more, talked more, she even sang along with the piano player when he came on Wednesdays. What a relief!' **Zack**

TIP: Having a carer present round the clock will be expensive, as the average cost is about £12-£20 per hour, depending where in the UK you live, and on the nature of your illness. If you want to spend your last weeks at home and can manage, as Sarah's father was able to, with six hours carer support a day, it might well be cheaper than going to a nursing home (c. £540 vs £860, for instance).

EXAMPLE 1

Dora has worsening dementia. She lives in a one-bedroom council flat and has fallen twice, badly bruising her hip. As a result of her sore leg, Dora is spending more of her time in bed, and is very frail. Social Services have been in contact with Dora's family, as Dora is no longer able to make decisions. There is no Power of Attorney (see Chapter 7), so the social worker takes charge of Dora's care needs and does a Needs Assessment. Alongside Dora's family, they have decided that she would benefit from having four care calls a day. As we have seen, this is the maximum amount of input that is available for care at home via Social Services.

Unfortunately, Dora's local care company are stretched and can only offer three visits per day, so her daughter has opted to come and see her mum every evening to make sure she is OK. Her daughter works 9-5, but luckily she lives nearby.

As Dora has some savings, she is paying for most of her care from them, but as Dora is over 65 she is entitled to Attendance Allowance, currently £83.10 per week, as she needs help both in the day and at night. Dora is currently likely to stay at home as she is spending most of her time in bed so is not at risk of falls or wandering out of her house.

5.2 Practical adaptations to make being at home easier

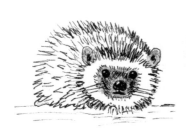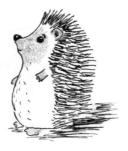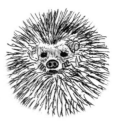

We are such resilient, adaptable creatures. Life throws problems at us and we bend our shape to try and accommodate them. But it isn't easy. Adapting to illness can require unexpected changes to our bodies, but also to our home life. As illness progresses, we tend to become more reliant on assistance. This can be help from a person, or it can be help from physical aids that aim to make life safer and easier.

Occupational Therapists (OTs), who we mentioned in 4.4, are ideally placed to help organise changes at home. They can come to visit, looking at the whole environment of your house and checking for fire hazards, especially heating and kitchen appliances. They can arrange mobility aids, commonly including:

- **Cutlery** – specially adapted to aid grip.
- **Grab rails** – these give you a sturdy rail or handle to hold onto so you can pull yourself up or safely sit down. They can be fitted along the stairs, at your front door steps, in your bath or shower or by the side of your bed – or in all of these places.
- **Stair lifts** – these can sometimes be hired rather than bought.
- **Hoists** – to enable movement from bed to chair and back again. Some areas organise these aids via the District Nursing service.
- **Walking aids** – from canes to frames.
- **Seat risers** – to make it easier to get out of a chair.
- **Loo seat risers** – so you don't sit so low and can get up from the toilet more easily.

TIP: A key safe can be attached to the wall outside your house. These are coded and contain the key to your front or back door for carers to gain entry or in case of emergency access needs. If you have a key safe, ensure that the right people have the code: your GP surgery, District Nurses, trusted neighbour.

There are a whole host of aids and adaptations available, so as you can see it's worthwhile ensuring you have contact with your local OT specialist. You can access them through your local Social Services, but if you have problems and need assistance urgently, do let your GP or District Nurse know, too, and they may be able to speed things along for you.

There is also general guidance around keeping safe at home from the Alzheimer's Society[18] website, which can be applied to any vulnerable person.

EXAMPLE 2

Getting upstairs can be tricky when you are less mobile. For Karen this was a real worry as she lived on her own. At 57 she was diagnosed with Motor Neurone Disease, which quickly affected her ability to walk. Her bedroom and bathroom were upstairs. After being assessed, Karen and her social worker organised:

- A key safe for the district nurses to easily access the house. They would call first to say they were on their way.
- A pendant alarm to wear on her wrist. If she had a fall she could push this button and help would be alerted.
- Hiring a stair lift. Karen knew she had an aggressive form of this disease and that the time ahead would be shorter than for other people. Rather than buying a stair lift she hired one for six months, whilst looking to find alternative accommodation all on one floor.
- Application for an electric wheelchair.
- Personal Independence Payment (PIPs).

Karen didn't need any carers to come and help her right away, but if things at home changed she had a social worker who knew her situation that she could contact quickly to get help.

For those with severe disabilities, or rapidly progressing disease, an application can be made for **Continuing Health Care funding (CHC)**. This means that your care is paid for by the Health Service rather than by Social Services, and is **free**. This can be incredibly helpful for those living with complex needs and limited resources. Application is a lengthy process and is often started by the District Nursing and Social Work team. Eligibility and access to this funding is restricted. There is more guidance here: www.nhs.uk/Conditions/social-care-and-support-guide/Pages/nhs-continuing-care.aspx

5.3 Co-ordinating care at home

As things change, there can be more complexity and so more need. This is when multiple services get involved. Let me explain how it fits together, again using an example:

EXAMPLE 3

Thomas has metastatic prostate cancer. His pain has worsened and he is getting very low in mood. He lives alone in a large house and has no carers. His Macmillan Nurse, Liz, has been to visit for the first time. Liz spends two hours with Thomas, going through all his issues. Together they make a plan to improve things at home:

- Increase pain relief by starting Morphine liquid at 5mg four hourly. Continue taking paracetamol, two tablets four times a day. Add in a laxative as the Morphine is constipating.
- Refer to the Day Hospice.
- Refer to Social Services to get an assessment for care at Thomas's home.
- Liaise with Thomas' GP to get the medication prescribed and to ask for a home visit for Thomas in the next few days to see how he is getting on.
- When they've done this, Liz asks Thomas, *'That's a lot to take in. Do you want me to write it down?'*
  'Oh yes,' says Thomas, *'I'll forget the moment you leave!'*
  Liz writes the plan down. *'Anything else on your mind?'*
  'No, no. That'll do. I'm tired now.'
  'OK,' says Liz. *'We can talk more next time. Maybe think about some of the things that matter to you in the future?'*
  'Having a good kip,' says Thomas, so Liz leaves it there for now.
- Liz arranges a follow up phone call to Thomas next week to see how he is doing and plans to come back in four weeks' time for a home visit.

- Two weeks later Thomas has a fall. He has cut his leg and calls Liz for help. She arranges for the District Nurse to visit to dress Thomas' wound. The District Nurse finds that Thomas has a small sore developing on his bottom

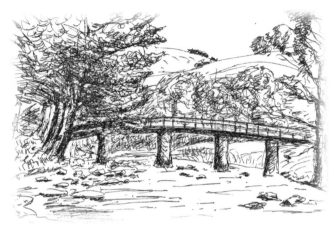

and so attends to this, as well as ordering a pressure-relieving mattress for him. The District Nurse also finds out that Social Services haven't been round yet, and calls them. She gets a definite date as to when they will come to see Thomas.

- Liz calls Thomas, who is feeling more comfortable now. The Morphine is helping his pain, and his sore bottom is getting better. He has had his first carer's visit, and likes one of them in particular as they can talk about going fishing.

For your own notes:

....

....

....

....

III. CARING FOR YOURSELF

6. YOUR PHYSICAL WELLBEING

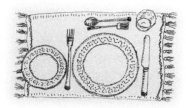

'I look at what she's made me for tea, and it looks lovely, and smells great. But I just can't face it. I take a bite and then I'm done.' **Philip, 71**

'"Go for a jog? Are you mad?" I said to her. But she was right. I got outside and took a few steps, went round the block, and I felt OK. I even slept that night for the first time in ages.' **Naz, 44**

In these changeable times it can be hard to imagine that there is much point in taking care of your body. But it's not really like that. As we have seen, people will live with life-shortening illnesses for a variable amount of time. As we don't know what lies ahead, it can make a real difference to look after yourself physically, enabling you to make the most of the day.

6.1 Food

I remember lazy hungover days, reaching for biscuits rather than cooking a meal. They seemed to help me feel better back then, but these days I'm not as robust, and it seems junk food isn't the cure it once was. One way of making the day ahead better is to make sure you eat well and stay properly hydrated. It may be tempting to think that because you have a life-shortening illness it doesn't matter what you eat or drink. But it can help. There are numerous diets advocated for improving health in life-limiting illnesses, and by all means have a look and try them. Here are some links to start you off:

- **Heart failure:** www.heart-failure.co.uk/living-with/ lifestyle-changes/diet/index.htm
- **Lung conditions:** www.blf.org.uk/support-for-you/eating-well/diet-and-my-symptoms
- **Cancers:** www.macmillan.org.uk/information-and-support/ coping/maintaining-a-healthy-lifestyle/healthy-eating
- **Kidney disease:** www.kidney.org/nutrition

The gist on all the websites is the same. Try to have a diet balanced with fruit and vegetables, watch your salt intake as this affects fluid balance, and watch your fat intake too. Increasing your fruit and veg consumption can help to reduce constipation, though conversely it can worsen diarrhoea. We'll look at some pharmaceutical options that can help to ease both of these in Chapter 9.

TIP: If your appetite is poor, or if you feel full easily, then eating smaller portions more often may be of benefit. Tangy sweets, chewing gum and pineapple chunks can help with a dry mouth.

There also comes a point when it's fine to eat what you fancy. Things aren't going to change, weight isn't going to be gained back.

Our loved ones are often very keen to feed us. It's a primal nurturing function, and it can be heart-breaking for them to see you not eat well.

TIP: If you're caring for someone, try a smaller plate with less food on it. Reducing expectations can help both of you feel less worried. A slice of cheese and a couple of crackers. A couple of

scoops of ice cream with a few grapes or cherries. Ice cream is very useful as it has lots of calories, and being cold can stimulate jaded taste buds.

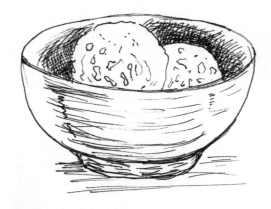

And there may be times you only want junk food and chocolate and wine, which is fine but may make you feel unwell in ways that you're not used to. Watch out for unexpected reactions with things like your painkillers; the combination of Morphine and alcohol will make you much more sleepy.

Eating can be especially difficult if you are feeling sick. We'll look at treating nausea and a dry mouth in Chapter 9. If things are particularly difficult, then the input of a dietician (see Chapter 4) can be useful.

TIP: It's worth pausing to check your medication: are you on too many tablets? Ask your doctor if you really need *everything* you have been prescribed. Some drugs can worsen nausea and constipation. Is it time to stop your statin? Is it time to stop your blood pressure medication? This can be difficult if you've been told to adhere to a drug regimen for a long time – but your team should be able to help you weigh up the risks versus the benefits of continuing all your prescriptions, particularly medication aimed at preventing future illness.

6.2 Fluids

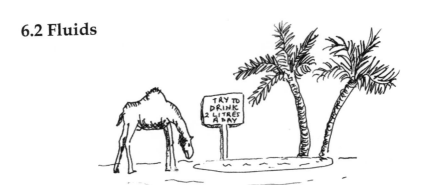

If you're weary, being asked to take another sip of water can be irritating. Swallowing large quantities of fluid can be a burden. On top of that, disease itself creates feelings of nausea too, putting you off drinking water. Fevers will worsen the situation due to sweating, as will some medications such as water tablets (diuretics).

TIP: To preserve your hydration try sipping water frequently, flavoured with cordials that have a good strong taste: lime or mint. Cold fizzy drinks can be more palatable. Drinking decaffeinated tea and coffee can help too, as can reducing your alcohol intake.

Dehydration can be picked up on blood tests, but signs to watch out for are:

- Increased confusion – feeling disorientated, not sure where you are or what is happening
- Increased tiredness – not being able to concentrate, more sleepy than usual
- Reduced passing of urine, with a darker colour
- Constipation

If you're concerned that you or your loved one is getting dehydrated, please contact your medical team. Things can deteriorate if left unattended, and you may be in need of intravenous fluids, which can sort the situation out quickly. I know this can mean a hospital admission – but sometimes all it takes is 24 hours of fluids and you can be back home again, feeling better, able to do a little more.

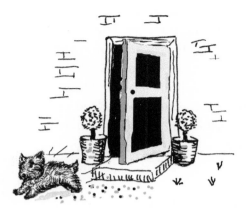

6.3 Exercise

As with diet, some exercise may help. This can be difficult to accept if you are feeling breathless or are in pain, but even though it sounds counter-intuitive, there is some evidence that keeping active during cancer treatment can improve the tiredness caused by your regimen. There are also exercise classes for people with COPD, even those who have quite severe disease.

Physiotherapy can also help: working together you can anticipate being a little more short of breath or in slightly more pain. Your physio should be able to reassure you that you're not causing damage by doing the activity. If you can trust that when you rest these feelings will pass, perhaps it will give you the confidence to do a little more. You may find you're surprised by the sense of wellbeing it can provide.

TIP: Doing some movement can also help to move your bowels.

Yes, those again! Never underestimate the irritation of constipation.

TIP: Have a go at doing what you can, but set a goal that is achievable. This may be a couple of lengths in the swimming pool, or it may be slowly walking into the kitchen to make a cup of tea and walking back to bed again.

Working with your physio and occupational therapists ,you'll get good advice on what exercise to do. They can also advise on making activities as safe as possible by suggesting adaptations to the way you perform tasks.

As with the dietary links above, there is sensible guidance available from the charities we've listed at the back of this book.

Here's an example to put the above into context:

EXAMPLE 1

You may recall Kenny, who has severe COPD – we met him in Chapter 2. Kenny coughs frequently. Kenny lives alone and sometimes finds it hard to motivate himself to cook properly for himself, so recently he has been losing weight.

Recently Kenny has been attending his local COPD physiotherapy programme, which runs for seven weeks. In Week 1, Kenny had his inhalers checked to make sure he is using them properly. His therapist has advised using a spacer device to help get more of the active ingredient into his lungs.

In Week 2 he was observed walking – he was grabbing onto the backs of chairs to stabilise himself – so a stick was suggested.

In Week 3, the physiotherapist watched Kenny coughing for most of the morning, and realised that he was bringing up a lot of mucous. She showed him how to take deeper breaths, and to cough more effectively so he could bring up more phlegm. She also suggested that Kenny spoke to his GP to see if he can be started on a drug called Carbocisteine, which can help loosen the phlegm and make it easier to cough up.

By Week 7, Kenny is more confident in his walking, he is getting more benefit from his inhalers, and his coughing has lessened. His GP (that's me) has also referred him to a dietician and he has put on a tiny bit of weight. I also stopped the medication that I was concerned may have been making Kenny feel worse.

Now Kenny is more stable, his medication seems to work a little better, and he is now able to walk to the shop on the corner on his own even though he still feels breathless. It's not a huge change, but

Kenny is not worrying so much about his breathing, and it means more independence and improved days. He quite likes the 'build-up' protein drinks the dietician recommended, but he prefers the fruit ones to the milkshakes. And he's really glad we stopped three of his tablets – he says he no longer feels as if he's rattling with pills.

6.4 Intimacy and sex

There will be times when you feel unwell and want to be left alone. You may have concerns that your treatment prevents you from close contact. I'd be very surprised if this was the case. However, you may not feel like it, which is a different matter. There will also be times that you may feel back to your normal self and want to be close to your partner. Sexuality can be central to our being, so if something is wrong or you are worrying, please ask. Physical contact is so important for us as humans – touching, stroking, kissing, hugging – these all form part of our world and shouldn't be ignored.

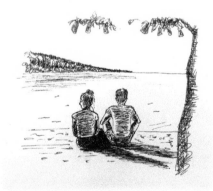

Straight or gay, do ask if anything is bothering you. For men, many medications can interfere with erections, but these can often be alleviated with drugs like Viagra (sildenafil). For women, medications can interfere with sexual drive and function too, but these can often be alleviated by lubricants – there's a huge range out there[19]. Your medical team is used to answering questions of any kind, and will try to help.

Please note: Pregnant women also can get serious illnesses. This is a specialised area requiring specialist input. Apart from all the general advice given here, the specific medication advice will very much depend on your circumstances, and your own medical team are best placed to help you make decisions around this difficult area.

6.5 Fatigue

Although we opened by talking about exercise as beneficial, sometimes illness causes overwhelming fatigue. Please be kind to yourself, and don't force yourself to do things that only cause you to feel more unwell. I suggest 'rest days' to patients with serious illness, to help them better manage the situation: if there is a day of activity coming up, then plan to rest the day before and/or the day after. This will give you time to recuperate and hopefully have more energy on the days when you need it. It means you can make a 'rest day' all about home comforts and indulgence, allowing yourself some time off.

6.6 Vaccination

If you are ill already, the last thing you need is another illness on top. Influenza is common in the autumn and winter months, and most strains can be prevented with vaccination.

TIP: Do get your flu jab. It's been shown to be the most effective intervention in COPD[20], even more so than stopping smoking.

Your doctor may also advise pneumococcal vaccination if you have recurrent chest infections. Please note: Shingles vaccine is a live vaccine and **not suitable** for anyone with compromised immunity such as those going through chemotherapy.

6.7 Physical changes during illness

Over time you will notice your body changing. Perhaps you don't have the energy you used to have. Doing the washing up is tiring, and you need someone else to do the garden work or vacuuming. It's OK. This is to be expected.

As diseases progress, they can make you tired and feel weak. It's a normal but frustrating part of what is happening to your body. Changing what we can expect of our bodies can be difficult. A climber will be used to high levels of fitness, a swimmer used to surging up and down the pool. Those of us who drive are used to hopping in the car and going where we want. But changes come, and gradually these freedoms aren't available. We can't climb, we can't swim, we can no longer drive. As our expectations of ourselves lessen, we can feel at a loss and hopeless.

6.8 When things get more difficult

Natural optimism can easily fail. Fatigue, loss of appetite, feeling more frail, all of these can contribute to making you feel low. Though the physical symptoms may settle with the medication your team prescribe, what about the feelings and worries you have? As with all life there are times when we get down, and sometimes this can be bad enough to interfere with our daily activities. (We look at this in more detail in Chapter 7).

If you are finding it hard to care for yourself alone, to feed yourself, and you're spending more time in bed than out of it, this can all indicate that time ahead may be getting quite short. Very few of us are ever ready to let go of life, and these changes can be deeply distressing and worrying. Check with your team that what is happening is in line with what they expect. It may be that something needs tweaking – anaemia can be treated with a transfusion, and sickness with medication for instance. Please ask, as they will do all they can to ensure you are as comfortable as possible.

'When I was eight, I saw a group of boys performing crazy postures on a beach in India. My aunt told me that being a girl, yoga was not for me. But I wanted to do it and I said, "If boys can do it, so can I. I am still proud of that body even though I have inoperable cancer. I am grateful for all it has given me.' **Tia, 96.**

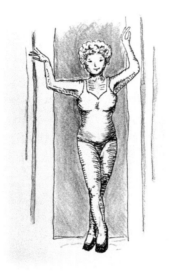

7. YOUR PSYCHOLOGICAL AND SPIRITUAL WELLBEING

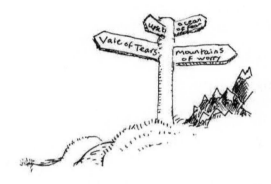

'I have a strong faith. When I lost my son my congregation helped me through it. Now that I'm ill myself, I turn to God for comfort.' **Alicia, 56**

'I don't believe in God or anything – though sometimes I wish I did – and when I got the diagnosis, it threw me hugely, and my depression came back with a jolt. I thought I'd beaten it years ago, but here were the old demons, screaming in my head. My GP spotted I was talking the way I had to her when I was really down before, and we talked about going back on medication. It helped a bit. Turned the volume down.' **Lee, 37**

We react to shocks and changes in our lives very differently, and this can depend much upon our circumstances. Being told that you have a life-shortening illness can leave you feeling bereft. Feelings of loss can come and go, and at times can be overwhelming. Some people struggle hugely not just with feeling unwell, but also with the idea of time running out and the consequences of diagnosis. It's as if you are already grieving for your own life. Others are pragmatic, and manage to detach themselves enough to plan their own funeral. (If the latter appeals to you, you'll find pointers in Chapter 12).

For many, depression and anxiety are ever-present. This is understandably common. You may already have been suffering from one or both of these, with the disease compounding them. As if being ill wasn't enough! Identifying that something is up can help to find a way forward. And the sooner the better. Let's look firstly at why these feelings may be happening.

7.1 Grieving an illness

If we look at the stages[21] of grief and loss as originally proposed by Elisabeth Kubler-Ross, these may help to explain some of what you are going through. Rather than feeling all at sea and wondering why, you might come to see what is happening is a normal part of the very difficult experience of living with a serious illness:

- **Shock** – being told you have a serious illness. Feeling overwhelmed and frightened.
- **Anger** – often a combination of frustration, fury, and confusion. How can this have happened? Why me? Why now?
- **Depression and detachment** – withdrawal, a desire to be alone in your suffering. This can combine with feelings of helplessness and isolation.
- **Bargaining** – on the journey to acceptance of what is happening there can be a desire to tell your own story, a wish to talk through the situation repeatedly, in the hope that some sense will emerge from the confusion.
- **Acceptance** – realisation that this is what is happening. Finding your own identity and meaning in your loss.

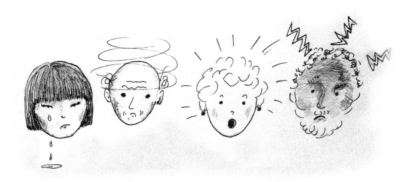

'Rather than seeing grief as a series of stages that we progress through step by step, it can be more helpful to see it like a piece of string or wool[22], that curls back round itself and intertwines,' says Sarah. 'Our emotions are not in any way fixed. We each go up, down, twist, turn and loop back and forth in our own unique fashion. Sometimes our string can get knotted, so we can experience several feelings all at once, which makes it very hard to unravel what's what.'

TIP: Grieving in illness means we can swing wildly from feelings of loss and despair to those of acceptance when the day feels bearable. Please know that this is normal, that this is OK, and it's usually what everyone is feeling even if they show it in their own different ways. We are such similar creatures, desiring calm and love in the chaotic currents of life.

If these feelings are interfering with your ability to function, upsetting your ability to make decisions or to find ways forward, then it is likely that you will need help. Psychological support comes in a variety of different levels, with or without medication. There should be psychological support close to you, often available at your local hospice.

TIP: Getting help early on should lessen the impact of depression and anxiety on your daily activities.

Changes to watch out for include:

- Feeling low
- Sleeping too little or too much
- Not being able to concentrate
- Eating too little or too much
- Talking too fast, or barely at all
- Feelings of panic and breathlessness
- Physical symptoms worsening – they can do this with stress and worry
- Withdrawing from friends and loved ones
- Cancelling outpatients appointments if you don't feel like going
- Avoiding going to work
- Thoughts of hurting yourself

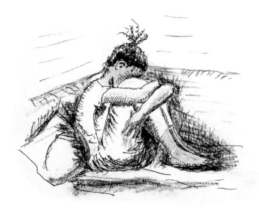

And then there is rage. Fury. We are programmed to live, no wonder we fight dying so hard. The common anger I see is around those who are dying whilst still young. It has no fairness to it, and life, with its pull to death, makes no sense. Why not be angry? Why not rage?

But if this anger is upsetting you and those around you, we do know that talking and talking and talking and being heard can help to bring moments of calm. It can't change the situation, it can't take the pain and awfulness away, but it can provide solace and acknowledgement.

For those who withdraw into themselves, the attempt to talk can be scary. **Find the one person you feel you can trust and let them have your thoughts**. You won't upset them, though they may cry with you. You may find someone who is there to help, to hold these harsh emotions with you. Please let them.

To feel some – or indeed all – of these things after diagnosis is, as I hope we've helped explain, completely understandable. But if you are suffering over a prolonged period (a good rule of thumb is more than two weeks) and especially if you are experiencing thoughts of suicide, then please do discuss your mood with your GP straight away.

7.2 Getting specialist help

7.2i Assessing mood

There are many tools used to measure your mood. One of the commoner tests is called the PHQ9 (Patient Health Questionnaire)[23], which asks about specific symptoms and how often you are feeling these. It helps to show how much impact your mood is having on your life: the higher the score, the greater the likelihood that support is needed.

Help can come in the form of talking, which can be talking to your loved ones or your doctor. You'll also find that almost every clinician who you come across in your palliative care experiences wants to talk. They'll be inquisitive about how you are physically, but many of us also want to know about how you are coping mentally. It's the remit of Macmillan Nurses, GPs, District Nurses and hospice staff to dig deeper and find out how things are going. They know how hard it can be. For some people this is enough, being reassured by the team. Hugging, crying, getting angry or withdrawn – however you respond to what is happening, we are human and feel empathy for what you are going through, and want to help alleviate that distress.

7.2ii Talking to a therapist or counsellor

Sometimes talking like this is not always enough. More time can be needed to deal with complex issues like:

- Struggling with a diagnosis
- Difficulty coping with the losses that illness brings
- Grieving for time ahead that will be lost, especially for those with young children
- A distraught partner, unable to face what is happening to you
- Feeling suicidal, that all hope is gone

And whilst we've devoted space here to mental wellbeing, a book can never be a substitute for seeing a counsellor in person, where you can talk and be individually supported. So if what I'm saying here resonates with you, then counselling is likely to not only help, but be needed, and I would strongly advise meeting with a counsellor sooner rather than later. This will give you time to explore the situation you are in and how you are reacting to it. The counsellor will work with you to find the best way forward, provide space to talk at length, and discuss strategies such as:

- Learning how to manage feelings of anxiety when panic rises
- Reflecting on and managing feelings of loss
- Living with an uncertain future
- Creating hope in difficult circumstances

Like all the areas we have looked at previously, this won't change the disease, or alter prognosis, but it can make the time ahead more bearable.

7.2iii Where to find a therapist or counsellor

There are therapists who are trained in supporting people with illness – they usually work in or are allied to your local hospice.

(Don't forget that hospices look after people with any life-limiting disease, not just cancer.) In addition, local cancer centres often have a psycho-oncology team, who can support people struggling emotionally with their cancer journey.

Alternatively, if you have the funds, you might decide to consult someone privately, as this might allow you to access a greater number of sessions. Finding someone reputable with experience of life-limiting illness is important, so ask around for recommendations, or look on Cruse, Dying Matters or The Priory Group websites[24].

'Some people worry that they're not going to connect with their therapist,' says Sarah. 'And sometimes you may not. But many therapists will be happy to start with just one session so you can get the measure of one another before committing to anything further, so don't let that fear put you off.'

7.2iv Medication

Medication is sometimes offered for anxiety and depression if it is deemed appropriate and safe in your situation. Drugs called SSRIs are commonly used first, and include Sertraline and Citalopram. Frustratingly, they can take two or more weeks to become effective, causing only side effects when first started. Given time, they should start to settle your mood, stopping the low times being so very low.

An alternative drug is Mirtazapine, which is also used for those struggling with sleep as it is sedating. It can stimulate appetite in some people, which is useful in serious illness when hunger seems to disappear.

Your doctor will go through the pros and cons of taking these medications, and their potential side effects. And please, if you have previously been prescribed these kinds of medications, do let your medical team know. If you notice changes happening to your mood, it may be useful to restart them sooner rather than later.

7.2v Complementary therapies

There is a wealth of non-medicinal help available too, including complementary therapies. Here are a few worth asking your Palliative Care Team about, as they may be available at your local hospice:

- **Reflexology** was documented by the Egyptians around 3000BC. It **involves using pressure points in the feet, each linked to a specific organ or system in the body, promoting positive energy flow.** Specific protocols are followed when treating different diseases, but this form of massage can be great for general relaxation too, helping to cope with the emotional impact of diagnosis. It promotes a sense of calm integration, and can help manage anxiety by reducing the impetus into fight-or-flight mode.
- **Meditation and relaxation.** Spending time with a therapist and concentrating on breathing and relaxing can help ease physical and mental symptoms of anxiety. This can also include Mindfulness techniques, which focus on living in the present moment and help to reduce stress and worry.
- **Massage.** Bringing feelings of relief and wellbeing.
- **Hydrotherapy.** Spending time in water, usually with a physiotherapist, can feel lovely. As water supports our bodies and 'lightens' our weight, it is easier to move sore limbs and do gentle exercise.
- **Acupuncture.** Acupuncture, an ancient Chinese medicine, involves the usually painless process of placing extremely

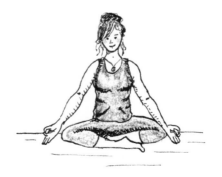

thin needles into the skin along specific 'acupuncture points'. The aim is to free up blocked channels, restore equilibrium and create a sense of calm.

- **Yoga.** The fundamentals of yoga are all about breathing, and if you're suffering from pain, fatigue or anxiety you may find it particularly beneficial. Some hospices offer specific yoga classes or sessions for patients focusing on pain management, for instance. A further advantage to yoga is that the practices, once learned, can be done at home on your own, and if you can't make it to a class or to a hospice session, 15 minutes of breathing exercises or just lying down focusing on the breath can work wonders.

'I've been to classes where where one person is literally lying down for most of it, but they are still getting some benefit.' **Pippa, 52**

Receiving kind, soothing therapies, with a gentle human touch, in a quiet safe space, can give wonderful feelings of wellbeing and warmth that can last for hours, sometimes days.

'I feel better about myself when my hair is set nicely. So once a fortnight a hairdresser comes to visit and does it for me.' **Hester, 83**

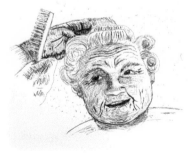

'Some people are sceptical about alternative treatments, but don't let that put you off: if one of these appeals to you, why not give it a try? After all, if a treatment or little bit of pampering improves how you feel either physically, mentally or both, then it's good news, because your overall wellbeing is the most important thing.' **Sarah**

'I don't want to talk about my disease. I find it too upsetting. But I go to the Day Hospice for the therapy in the afternoon, and come home feeling like some of the weight of my heavy body has been lifted. It's what I really enjoy.' **Jeremiah, 49**

7.2vi Books that may help

There are many supportive books available to help you better understand your emotional journey. Have a look at the Bibliography section at the end of this book. There are two books in this series that may help if depression and/or anxiety are causing distress – *Making Friends with Anxiety* and *Making Friends with Depression*[25]. In them Sarah explores the feelings of anxiety and depression, and many of the treatments we've touched on here in more detail. There is also a support group on Facebook, which you can find here: facebook.com/ groups/makingfriendswithanxiety and are welcome to join.

7.3 Spiritual Support

We live in more secular times, but how we experience the world and how we interpret the unexplained is wildly and gloriously various. Both Sarah and I feel that whatever brings comfort as opposed to distress is the way forward. This may be simple prayer time whilst on your own, with your faith leader or family, or it may be an important ritual that you wish to fulfil.

'When my stepfather, Adrian, was told he had cancer and that it would, ultimately, be terminal, the first thing he did on return from seeing the consultant was to walk up to the village church, discuss it with the vicar and book his burial spot. He wanted to make sure his grave was in the grounds of the place of worship that meant a lot to him. When he came back he told my mum and me what he'd done. "I also got a haircut," he added. That he'd stopped off at the village barber on the way home still makes me smile. That mix of pragmatism and spiritual belief was Adrian to a T.' **Sarah**

102

If faith is central to your life, as it was to Sarah's stepfather, let your Palliative Care Team know. Don't forget that the team includes your GP and District Nurse. They won't guess or assume on matters of faith. There are certain tenets of faith that are vital to some – being attended to by only one gender or being able to pray frequently. Your team will aim to facilitate whatever is needed.

I had a patient who wanted to spend his last days in Pakistan. He was very ill, requiring oxygen and Morphine. He was adamant he wanted to fly home, and with his family we managed to get an airline to take him in his poorly condition, as they understood the importance of his request. We organised transport to the airport via ambulance, organised documents for the Controlled Drugs medication, and off he went, dying only a few days later where he wished to be. It can't always be done, but if your wish isn't known then it won't happen.

Atheist or agnostic patients may gain comfort from making their own kind of ritual. My ritual is to sometimes light a candle and spend 10 quiet minutes listening to the surroundings, and then blowing the candle out. A ritual can be a gift to yourself, alone or with loved ones, treasuring that moment. It can be a simple thing like meditation, or a decorative event with chanting, dancing and poetry. The most important aspect is that it chimes with how you are feeling, making it a special time for you.

7.4 Coping with work

If your professional life means a lot to you, you may wish to carry on working, even though you know that your time left is limited.

'Work is a pleasurable activity for some of us,' says Sarah. 'It can help take your mind off your circumstance and give you a sense of purpose. Think of Matisse! He created some of his best-known art in the final decade of his life, observing "I have needed all that time to reach the stage where I can say what I want to say", even though, following surgeries for cancer of the intestine, he was mostly confined to his bed and a wheelchair. His movement was limited so he pared back to the simplest materials – coloured paper and scissors, just as a child might use. He described his collages as "drawing with scissors", but what a gift his cut outs were to the world. Admittedly he had a full-time assistant[26] which most of us don't, but by taking regular breaks perhaps you can keep your hand in, which may lift your spirits if you love your work.'

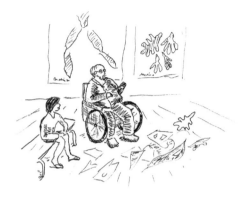

There is more practical information on work, sick notes, and the legal aspects of working with a disability in Chapter 10.

7.5 Holidays – taking a break from treatment

Holidays are there for pleasure and a break from the ordinary pressures of life. The same is true of treatment: there will be times you want a break from all that's going on. Planning your holiday around treatment regimens is really important, ensuring that you're safe to travel, that you're not missing courses of medication, and that your health team know where you are if they need to get in touch with you. Liaising with the hospital will ensure that you do this at the right time, with everyone aware of your plan of care.

> **FACT: Insurance can be a real problem for someone living with a life-limiting illness. Will your insurance cover you for the country you are visiting? It's worth shopping around for quotes, as you will be surprised the difference between companies. It's worth contacting the charity appropriate to your illness, as they are often up to date on where to find better deals.**

This means it's easier to travel within the UK, but it doesn't mean you are confined to it. If you want to go abroad, here are some things to think about:

- How long is the travel time? Will you need access to medication during travel? Do you need to have blood thinners if you're going to be sitting still for a long time? (Flights to and from Australia, the Far East and the Americas spring to mind.)
- If you are travelling abroad with controlled drugs like Morphine, you will need paperwork to pass through customs more easily[27].
- If something happened abroad, would you want care there or back at home? And, though hard to imagine, what about if you die whilst abroad? Would you want someone to bring your body home? Repatriation of a body can be very expensive. These are such hard things to think about, but a discussion with your medical team should help make the issues clearer.

7.6 Creating hope

It's odd to talk of hope, perhaps, but we spend most of the time living deep within the realms of hope. Why not now, even if time is shortening? In illness too, there is a need for hope. We can hope the day is untroubled, that we'll achieve a tricky task, that someone will behave kindly towards us. Today may feel better than yesterday. Tomorrow may be even better than that. When the medication kicks in, it's reasonable to hope that you will feel a bit better physically, which may lift mood.

Planning something to look forward to can help to plant a seed of hope too. Think of something achievable that you might like to do today, even if it's planning a day in bed. Then think of something for the weekend ahead. Perhaps a little like this:

- Today I'm going to treat myself to a day in bed.
- Today I'm going to meet my friend in the pub, even if I only drink fizzy water.

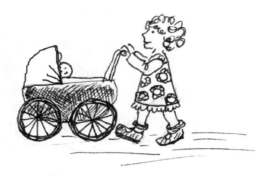

- On Saturday, if I feel OK, I'm going to meet my friend for a cup of tea. And if I'm really feeling OK then we might go to the cinema.
- Next month I'd really like to go to the seaside for the day. Or to the countryside to a favourite picnic spot. Put it in your diary.
- Anniversaries – it's my daughter's birthday in September. I'd really like to make the effort to go and stay with her and my granddaughter, even though they are in Germany. Maybe for a week. Maybe for a weekend.

Putting dates like these in your diary can create things to look forward to, hope as well as distraction. Even events that aren't welcome – a third course of chemotherapy – can have a different slant with some planning. How about stopping somewhere you like on the way home from the hospital for a break? That way it's not just the journey there and back again. A woodland walk, a browse in a local shop, a trip to the viewing point at the local airport! I wonder what you would like to do?

IV. TREATMENTS

8. MEDICAL TREATMENTS

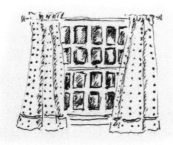

'I'll have whatever's offered. I'm too young to die. I'll try anything.'
Jim, 32 – oral cancer

'Can't I have a transplant? Why can't they give me a new set of lungs?' **Jeff, 77 – COPD**

Let's take a look at potential medical treatments in life-shortening illnesses. It may seem odd to think of treatments in this setting, but if you think that **the aim is to manage and hopefully reduce the impact on daily living caused by the disease,** then perhaps it makes more sense. In this chapter we'll focus on interventions aimed at slowing the disease processes down. In the next chapter we'll be looking at supportive care for symptoms you may be suffering. Feel free to skip forwards if this is the information you need right now.

In a moment, we'll take a brief look at some of the commoner diseases and their treatment, but we can look at some general principles of care. **For any disease, the supportive teams are looking to provide both increased quality and quantity of life**. For the majority of non-cancer diseases doctors will rely on medication to control physical symptoms. Heart patients will need tablets to optimise the heart's function, and respiratory patients may need steroids, antibiotics and inhalers to help them breathe more easily and we'll look at these in the second half of the chapter. If you have cancer, you may think that aggressive treatment suits your situation best, or you may think the exact opposite, wishing to spend any time ahead at home and avoiding potential side effects. Perhaps both are possible, or somewhere in between.

TIP: Stay in touch with your GP surgery.

Before we look at hospital treatments, do remember that your GP surgery is there for you throughout. Even though you are under the care of the hospital, they can help with side effects of treatment. They can issue medications for nausea, sickness and constipation, as well as for pain. **Prescriptions are free for those having cancer treatment. Your GP surgery can provide free prescription application forms, Fit Notes, and administer vaccinations** (all of which we touched on in Chapter 5), **and even more importantly, talk to you**. Your GP is there to discuss how it's going, what's working and what isn't. We are usually a compassionate bunch of people who want you to have as easy a time as possible.

Medical treatments offered will be particular to your situation, so **two people with exactly the same disease may be offered different regimens**. It will depend on factors such as how well you are, what else you may be suffering from, and what your wishes might be. If you're concerned you're not getting the right treatment for you, do ask your team. They should be able to explain their decisions to you, or fix any mistakes.

8.1 Options in Cancer

Which treatment may help you will vary, depending on the type and stage of your illness. For some cancer patients there is a clear route:

surgery to remove a lump, followed by radiotherapy to the area, and/or chemotherapy to mop up cells that may have spread. Even if the cancer has advanced and there isn't a chance of cure, these measures can still sometimes help you to feel better, and possibly live longer, by slowing the disease down. Even though they may be widespread, if the cancer cells have certain traits, they may be sensitive to hormone therapy and lie dormant for some time ahead.

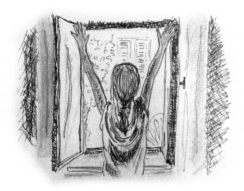

'I had metastatic disease when I was diagnosed, but the chemo worked really well. After three months it had all shrunk down and I felt back to my normal self.' **Debbie, 44, breast cancer**

8.1i Surgery

The aim of surgery is to remove abnormal tissue that is interfering with the normal functioning of the body. This can range from taking out a brain tumour, trying to maintain language and mobility, to removing a colon cancer that is blocking the bowel. Unblocking the bowel may not remove all the cancer cells but it can return the bowel to normal function allowing you to get on with life without pain and sickness.

'I've had this for two years. I just can't stand it any more. Why can't they take it out of me?' **Ellen, 78, bladder cancer**

Surgery is not always an option if the risks outweigh the benefits. Some patients are too poorly, and some cancers are too widespread (the medical word is 'disseminated' or 'metastatic' in case you hear the doctors chatting). It may seem very strange that a small tumour can't be removed but this will be because it is just not safe. It may be because the tumour is located in a difficult place to reach. It may be because the tumour is in several places or attached to another organ, and the surgeon won't be able to get in there.

Your team will explain the benefits versus the risks of surgery, and together you can decide the best way forward, though this isn't always an easy clear cut decision.

TIP: Do take your time. Doctors can make decisions quickly, but if you need time to think things through and discuss with your loved ones, then you can. My advice would be: tell the doctor you need time to think it through, and you can call his secretary with your decision. This may not be convenient for the doctor, but really, this is about you!

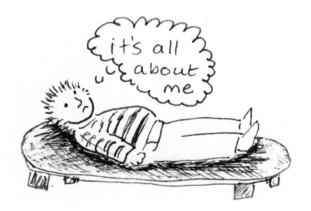

8.1ii Chemotherapy

Our cells are constantly being replaced, and this is a natural turnover. You'll see it every day with normal hair loss and skin flaking off. However, if this process gets out of control, then cancer cells can start to grow. Chemotherapy is a broad term used to describe a huge array of medications aimed at interfering with the ways cells replicate. It aims to allow normal cells to continue to grow, and interfere with cancerous ones.

The way people experience chemotherapy is a wide spread from good to bad:

'I felt nothing. Even my hair stayed in place. I can't believe it, the cancer has receded and I may have another year to see my grandchild grow.' **Carol, 62 – lung cancer**

'I was so sick. Sick, sick, sick. I wish I'd known how unwell I was going to be, I wouldn't have had it.' **John, 54 – breast cancer**

Which chemotherapy agent is used will depend on the cancer type, on how well you are, and what is available. There are common treatment regimens which are used as a first line, second line medications are used if the usual one hasn't worked, and then there are new trial drugs, which you may be offered if standard treatment isn't working.

Most cancer services are well equipped to explain why they are offering a certain regimen. They will give you written information about what the drugs are, what they do, and what the side effects might be. As these drugs interfere with normal cell activity, they also affect normal function, so common side effects include diarrhoea, hair loss, nausea and infection. Your immune system will be dampened down to try to kill the cancer cells. This means you will be more susceptible to infections. For some treatment regimens this is more likely than others. The staff are very used to dealing with the side effects: if you are suffering, do let them know as there may be a simple medication that helps your situation.

It can be hard to decide if you want to go through with chemotherapy. As we've seen previously, some people are really up for any treatment, and others find the prospect worrisome. It's OK to take a bit of time to mull things over. Waiting a few days to a couple of weeks may be alright, but check with your team as they will be able to better explain the consequences of holding back.

Chemotherapy is often given in 'cycles'. This means that you receive doses of the medication, then have a break whilst it does its work. You may be offered a number of cycles at the beginning, but find this number is adjusted according to how you respond. Don't worry, this is normal! Holding back on chemotherapy if you are unwell is reasonable, as it can be toxic. Having a break or even stopping midway through cycles means the team are looking after you and not taking risks with your health.

There are times you can be sitting in the waiting room, chatting to other patients with the same disease as you, but find out that they are getting quite a different treatment regimen to you. If you feel you aren't getting the right chemotherapy, or enough of it, then ask the Consultant or Clinical Nurse Specialist. They should be able to explain their rationale. Sometimes the decisions are really hard to make. The team have to weigh up the degree of your illness versus the potential harm of the medication.

8.1iii Radiotherapy

'I got sudden back pain and my legs went numb. I phoned the GP and within hours I was scanned, had a shot of radiotherapy, and now my legs are OK and my pain has gone. I can't believe how quickly it happened. I can't thank them enough.' **Jim, 76 – prostate cancer**

'I had diarrhoea for three weeks. It hurt to go to the loo, it hurt to pee, I lost control and was incontinent. But as they said, six weeks down the line I'm OK. I'm back to where I was, if a bit more tired.' **Mohammed, 78 – prostate cancer**

This extraordinary and painless technique, discovered by Marie Curie, is used to direct radiation in an accurate beam onto cancer cells in order to kill them. The aim is to reduce the size of the tumour and its local effects. As tumours grow, they can push on other nearby structures interfering with how they work. Imagine a lung cancer pushing on the airways, with radiotherapy aiming to open them up.

It's also useful if there are spinal tumours pushing on the spinal cord: these tumours can cause pain, weakness in the legs, and potentially incontinence too, as the nerves that control the bowel and bladder come from here. A single shot of radiation is sometimes enough to shrink the tumour down to allow normal function to resume and reduce pain from tumour pressure.

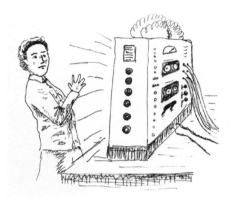

The type of machine, the duration of treatment, and the intensity of the radiation is decided by your oncologist. This can vary from one dose, to many doses over several weeks. Whilst you can rest assured radiotherapy machines do *not* look like Sarah's sci-fi illustration, some people do find them big, noisy and daunting at first. But, as with any new experience, familiarity should help to settle you in. The staff are skilled and know how to support you through this. And as with all aspects of your care, if you're unsure what is happening, please ask. Most people are really helpful and want to support you on your journey. They will emphasise that keeping still is important so that the beam is accurate. They will check on a regular basis that you're comfortable and doing OK.

Though it is painless at the time, side effects will develop afterwards, and these depend on the location, dose and duration of radiation. The more radiation you have, the more potential damage to local healthy tissue. Common effects include:

- Burns to the surrounding skin, which can be like sunburn. It's usually mild and treated with moisturising cream.

- Irritation to normal tissue at the site of the tumour. In pelvic cancers the sensitive bowel and bladder can be sore, leading to usually temporary pains on peeing and pooing. In head cancers this can impinge on swallowing – it's usual to prescribe liquid build-up drinks to keep your nutrition up.
- It's really common to feel tired after treatment. We looked at fatigue in Chapter 7, so have a re-read of that if you are experiencing this.

TIP: Whilst receiving treatment, it's quite normal to feel exhausted after doing even small activities. Make allowances for treatment days and the weeks afterwards, for that's when you're likely to be most tired – planning rest days can make the process easier.

Your energy levels should return a few weeks after the radio-therapy stops, depending on the stage of your disease.

8.2 Options in heart failure

The heart is a complex pump, taking blood with oxygen from the lungs and pumping it into the arteries for use around the body. Once the oxygen is delivered to the organs and tissues, blood returns to the heart to be pumped back into the lungs, and so on. This happens every second of our lives. When the heart isn't pumping well it is known as heart failure (a typically upsetting descriptive term from the medical profession for which I can only apologise!). As with any pump, when fluid gets stuck it pools, it splutters, and becomes inefficient. You'll know this from seeing an old car jerking along the road with a temperamental fuel or exhaust pipe. If oxygen doesn't easily get to the tissue that needs it, the body compensates by making you breathe faster, increasing your heart rate, and making you feel tired.

Heart failure symptoms are characterised by increasing breathlessness, pooling of fluid in the limbs and chest, and sometimes chest pain (angina) as the heart muscle, lacking oxygen, aches. The mainstay of treatment is to try to improve the machine.

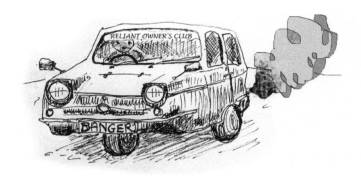

Here's what the medical team aim to do:

- Keep the heart pumping in as normal a rhythm as possible, usually by using a drug called a Beta Blocker (Bisoprolol is common), or implanting a pacemaker.
- Reduce swelling (called oedema). Swollen ankles and legs are the common indicator that the fluid is accumulating. By shifting fluid that has leaked into the soft tissues and skin back into the circulation, this swelling can be reduced. The mainstay of drugs are 'water tablets' or diuretics, usually Furosemide or Bumetanide.
- Control high blood pressure, aiming for readings around 130/80. Some cardiologists will aim for even lower blood pressures. Lots of different tablets can do this, including drugs like Ramipril, Losartan, and Amlodipine. There are wide ranges of medications similar to these three drugs, and if you have heart failure you are likely to be on one or more of them.
- Reduce and, if possible, stop angina by using drugs that dilate the arteries around the heart. These include Isosorbide Mononitrate (ISMN), Glyceryl Trinitrate (GTN) sprays or tablets under the tongue, Nicorandil, Ivabradine and Ranolizine.
- Morphine is useful too, as it helps by both reducing breathlessness and relieving angina.
- Education around managing breathlessness and fatigue helps to reduce these incapacitating symptoms.

The Heart Failure CNSs are skilled at getting the right balance of these different medications. As you can see from the list there are a lot to choose from, and making people feel better takes monitoring and frequent reviews. If the medications become less effective over time then other measures can be utilised, and we'll explore these in the next chapter.

EXAMPLE 1

John is 66 and had a heart attack six months ago. He hasn't made a good recovery as a lot of the heart muscle was damaged. He spends much of his time with his feet up, as his legs are swollen. Maxine, the Community Matron, took bloods yesterday and noticed that John's kidney function has worsened slightly. So she visits today. John is feeling OK, and his legs are less swollen than they have been for a while. So she reduces the dose of his water tablet, Bumetanide, as this may be working too hard and putting a strain on the kidneys. John is also complaining of breathlessness. She checks his oxygen levels with a finger probe and they are quite low. After chatting to John, he agrees to an assessment for oxygen as this may help his breathing. They talk more:

'John, things seem to be changing, don't you think?'

'I suppose. I'm more breathless. Legs are better though, aren't they?'

'Yes, today they look good. But I'm seeing you more often, and we're changing medication more frequently.'

'Mm.'

'One of the things we could do for your breathing would be to get you to a breathlessness course.'

'What's that?'

'It's a course at the local hospice, where they teach you breathing techniques and relaxation so you feel less bothered by your breathing.'

'I haven't got cancer, have I?'

'No, but the hospice looks after people with any kind of serious disease. Have a think and let me know. I'll be back next week to get some more blood off you and make sure your kidneys are OK and your legs aren't swelling up again."

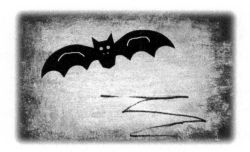

'*Vampire!*' says John. Then he agrees to attend the course at the day hospice and, in the end, it turns out that he enjoys it.

'*It was good to get out of the house,*' he says. '*Chance to meet some others who feel as bad as me.*'

8.3 Options in COPD

'*I can feel like I'm drowning, like I won't get my next breath in. It's horrible. Then the nurse comes, changes one thing, and I feel better for a while.*' **Jack, 62 – COPD**

Lungs rely on flexibility to rise and fall in normal breathing. As they stiffen with lung diseases they, like the heart, become less efficient at exchanging carbon dioxide for refreshing oxygen. The result is breathlessness, which can increase on doing normal activity. Along with breathlessness there is persistent coughing, coughing up sputum, and sometimes pain and sleeplessness from both of these. Weight loss is common as the disease progresses, and along with this comes fatigue. Anxiety and depression commonly occur too. All really frustrating.

There are several kinds of medication that work on lung tissue, aiming to improve its flexibility. The majority are inhalers – in different colours and shapes. The tricky things is knowing how to use them most effectively and also being aware when they have run out. Your GP practice nurse and Respiratory Clinical Nurse Specialist (CNS) are the health professionals best placed to help in the first instance. They can show you how to use your inhaler properly and ensure it's the best device for you. As things change more input from the respiratory CNS can help. Common medications include:

- Short-acting bronchodilators (SABAs) like Salbutamol/ Ventolin. This is the BLUE inhaler. It works quickly, but not for long. It's best used through a chamber or spacer device to ensure you're getting the full benefit.
- Long-acting bronchodilators (LABAs) – there are many! They include drugs like Salmeterol and Formeterol. They are usually given twice daily.
- Long-acting muscarinic antagnosists (LAMAs) – there are many! They include drugs like Tiotropium and Glycopyrrhonium. They are usually given once daily.
- LABA/LAMAs – these are combination inhalers of both the inhaler ingredients above. The idea is that they work together on different receptors in the lung at the same time. If given in one inhaler it means less work for you.
- Inhaled Corticosteroids (ICSs) – these are the mainstay of asthma control, and are also used in COPD when LABA/LAMA isn't enough or if you've needed steroid tablets for infections. The steroids reduce the inflammation in the lung tissue, reducing wheeze and constriction.
- LABA/LAMA/ICS – this will be in two inhalers to provide all the medication available in an inhaler to best optimise the situation.
- Carbocisteine – this is a mucolytic, a drug that liquefies sputum hopefully making it easier to cough up. If you're coughing up a lot of sticky phlegm this can be a great help.
- Nebulisers – these are pumps that force air through liquid medication, creating droplets that can be inhaled via a mask. Medication can include Salbutamol which opens up the airways as above, and also saline (salt water), which can help to loosen phlegm and make it easier to cough up.
- Oxygen – oxygen is useful in certain types of lung disease, but not all. Your team will decide if it suits your situation and will organise an assessment if your blood oxygen levels dip. Oxygen doesn't really work for breathlessness unless your oxygen levels are very low. Instead, there is good evidence for the use of hand held fans to bring relief.

- NIV (non-invasive ventilation) – in certain situations, when breathing becomes laboured, there are machines that can help to keep the airways open and push air into the lungs. Though they are noisy and usually require a tight mask to be worn over the nose and mouth, they can provide relief from some types of breathlessness.
- Antibiotics and steroids are used to control flare-ups of infections and wheezing. You may have a stock of these at home, called Rescue Packs, in case you keep having repeated problems. Long-term use of both medications can cause more harm than good but, again, it's about weighing the balance of risk versus benefits and this will be an individual decision based on each person's circumstances. Your medical team will help with this, ensuring you have the least medication for the best outcome.

Unfortunately, there are other lung diseases that don't respond well to inhalers, including pulmonary fibrosis and cystic fibrosis. They can be frustrating to treat, but the aim, as with heart failure, is to optimise your medication so that you are best able to do the things you want to do, such as having a shower, or taking your dog for a short walk. Your respiratory team may offer more experimental treatment aiming at slowing down these disease processes.

You'll find resources for these two conditions on p.198 at the back of this book.

EXAMPLE 2

Brenda has had COPD for 15 years now. She has lost a lot of weight recently and been into hospital twice for chest infections. Her respiratory nurse, Jan, has come round to check on things:

'I feel bad again,' says Brenda.

'In what way?' asks Jan.

'Coughing up muck, can't do anything, too breathless.'

Jan checks Brenda's chest. It sounds really noisy again. Her oxygen levels are lower than normal, at 87%.

'I think you've got another infection.'

'Oh no. Does that mean hospital?'

'No, I think we can try to manage it here. Have you got your Rescue Pack?'

'Yes, it's there by the fags.'

'Oh you're not smoking again are you!? OK, start the antibiotics and steroids today. Here, I'll help you. But before we do that, show me how you use your inhaler again.' Jan sees that Brenda is struggling with her inhaler, and decides to change the type to one Brenda can use with less effort. *'OK I'll call tomorrow and see how you've got on.'*

Jan helps Brenda to avoid another hospital admission. She calls the GP with the changes and to update them. The GP agrees to a joint visit the following week as things seem to be getting more difficult for Brenda, and they need to start discussions around her future care.

8.4 Options in neurological disease

'I put the mask on at night. It took ages to get used to it, but now I can sleep through, and I don't wake up that breathless or with a headache'. **Aisha, 55 – Motor Neurone Disease**

Neurological diseases, such as Parkinson's Disease, Huntington's Chorea and Motor Neurone Disease (MND) are characterised by increasingly poor functioning of the nervous system. Symptoms vary hugely, but the general trend is that they tend to worsen over time at different rates, so there is a lot of variety from person to person, case to case. This means one person with MND might have difficulty using their hands as these are the nerves that are affected, whilst someone else with MND might have problems with swallowing or speech instead. Your neurologist doctor will usually be a specialist in the disease type and be able to give clearer individual guidance on your situation and what can be expected as time passes. Things you might want to ask could be:

- Will this affect my ability to drive or work?
- How long will it take for me to notice changes?

- Is there a specific medication for my disease type?
- Is there a genetic part here – do I need to let my family know so they can get checked?
- Where can I get help for my individual problems?

One of the frustrations in neurological diseases is that there isn't a wealth of medication out there like there is for heart and lung diseases because the nervous system is harder to access and manipulate. This means medication can't stop the changes happening but it can either reduce symptoms or slow the speed of deterioration. Drugs like L-Dopa (Sinemet and Madopar) can ease Parkinson's disease symptoms, reducing rigidity and tremor, improving mobility. Riluzole is a drug used in Motor Neurone Disease, as it has been shown to improve prognosis a little.

The mainstay of caring for people with these progressive neurological conditions is to use any available medication, and then manage any physical, emotional or psychological symptoms as they arise on an individual basis. You may find there is help from an extended team of specialists who work alongside the doctors, including physiotherapists, occupational therapists, speech and language therapists (SALT team) and psychologists who specialise in a disease type.

Early intervention from the palliative and supportive care teams can also be of great benefit. Following assessments of the person's whole needs, from their physical symptoms to their home situation to their hopes and desires, a management plan can be formulated that addresses the issues that are causing trouble. We'll look at this in greater detail in Chapter 10.

EXAMPLE 3

Aisha has MND. She was diagnosed three years ago, and is now having more difficulty with her speech and breathing. Her legs are OK, but she is too breathless to walk any distance. Despite taking Riluzole, her MND has progressed to the point where she needs a lot of help to look after herself. Her GP visits:

'Hi Aisha, how are you doing?'

'Well, I'm in a bit of a rut.'

'In what way? Have things changed?'

'They're always changing. Every day I can feel my breathing get weaker.'

'Tell me about how you are managing your days.'

'Oh, it's so predictable! My day goes like this. Ali gets me up and helps me get dressed. It takes ages. He has to take off the NIV machine, then we slowly put on my clothes, resting every thirty seconds for me to get my breath back. He then goes off to work and Lily, the carer, arrives. She sorts out breakfast and medication – if I can be bothered to eat – and we have a chat about what's been going on. She's only there for 30 minutes, and she comes back at 12, then again at four. Between those times I'm usually on my own, watching telly, trying to read. I end up dozing all the time. It's really boring!'

'Does anyone else come to visit?'

'Charlotte, the Occupational Therapist lady, has been. She's asked if now is the right time for Ali to stop work to look after me. I can't ask him to do that! But I don't want to go into a home. It's really hard! And boring!'

'I'm so sorry, Aisha. Things seem more difficult. Perhaps it would be good if the Macmillan nurse came by again to talk through things with you?'

'Yeah, she was nice. Can you do that?'

'Of course. What are you doing tomorrow?'

'I'm off to the day hospice. I'm seeing the Reiki therapist. She's fantastic! I come out feeling really chilled. And Zara, my daughter, is coming over at the weekend with her baby boys. Twins! I can't wait to see them.'

'OK. I'll get the Macmillan nurse to call you to set a time, and then I'll come back in a couple of weeks and see how things are going. Have a nice weekend with Zara!'

'Thanks, doctor. See you soon.'

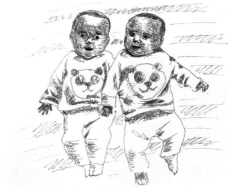

8.5 Options in dementia

It can be such a bombshell to be told that you or your loved one has dementia. Our minds spring forward, thinking of times of frailty that may lie ahead. Though the disease can't be stopped, being as ready as you can for what may lie ahead can make the journey easier to live with and easier to bear.

One of the key points is to get an early diagnosis. This can prompt the start of medication to try to slow down disease processes, and it can also trigger access to help such as an assessment by Social Services. Here are a few pointers to try to make the time ahead less worrying:

- **Early Diagnosis.** If you feel your memory isn't as sharp as it was, do see your GP to have it tested. There are a variety of memory tests they use. They use them repeatedly to see how things are going and if things are changing. It may seem insulting at first, being asked for things like your birthdate or your address, but the tests have been developed to assess small changes. Please bear with the questioner! If dementia is felt to be a possibility, your GP will refer you to a Memory Clinic, run by the Psychiatry Team. Here they will do more memory tests, and also organise a CT scan of your brain to make sure nothing else is causing the changes. You will also have blood tests to make sure nothing else is contributing to how you feel.
- **Medication.** Once a diagnosis is established, medication can be started, if appropriate. These medications aim to slow down the dementia process, though unfortunately not in all types of dementia. For example, they don't tend to work where the dementia is caused by poor blood supply to the brain, known as vascular dementia, nor in Lewy Body dementia associated with Parkinson's Disease.
- **Anticipation.** One of the most important things, in my experience, is to know what your wishes are whilst you have the facility to explain this clearly. You can do this in a number of ways, including The Advance Care Plan we discussed in

Chapter 1, where you put into writing what you may or may not want to happen in the future. Sharing this information with those close to you helps with any decisions that need to be made in the future. This is especially true if you are no longer able to make decisions for yourself.

- **Crisis minimisation.** Another part of anticipation is trying to head off any crisis. If you are concerned that you are becoming more unwell or unsafe, then do let those who help care for you know. Equally, if you are a carer and notice changes like this, then discuss it with all those involved so help can be put in place sooner rather than later.

Ensuring adequate care and support in the home environment is vital to having a safe and comfortable time ahead. This usually means having a Social Services assessment, or even a reassessment as things change, as we discussed in Chapter 5. **Once an assessment has happened, there will be a record of your case at the local Social Services office. This means that if an increase in care is needed it can be done more quickly as you are already known to the service.**

Looking after someone with dementia can be challenging, and the carers and loved ones doing this work can also need help and support, as we touched on in Chapter 3. Don't forget there is support available at Carers UK 0808 808 7777 carersuk.org and you can also find advice at alzheimers.org.uk.

8.6 Other disease groups

And what about the rest of the people with diseases not mentioned above? Our experiences show that there are as many different stories to tell about illness and suffering as there are people in the world. I still come across people suffering from conditions I've never heard of. This used to make me worry, rushing to textbooks to find out more about the disease process – what is it, what causes it, what can I do about it? That's fine if the condition is curable, but if it has no cure then the principles of palliative and supportive care work regardless. Why? Because the focus is about what the patient is experiencing, how they are coping, where they live and who is around to help. It's about how their worries, hopes and beliefs inform all of this, and how those working with a patient can ease the situation from day to day.

TIP: There can be too many drugs that do too many things, making you feel even more unwell. It's called polypharmacy. Ask your medical team if you need all the medication you are taking. For instance, do you need that statin, do you need those blood pressure tablets, do you need all of the painkillers you are taking?

8.7 Some general medical aids explained

There are devices designed to make life easier, or as necessity after certain operations. But their names can have a stigma attached. Often because it's not clear what they do, or they are linked to our waste elimination functions.

- **What is a catheter?** A catheter is a tube passed into the bladder to allow urine to flow into a connecting bag. It is used when people are too frail to get out of bed to use the toilet, or if there is no control over flow, causing constant leakage. Catheters can provide a solution to flow problems, but they are also implicated with infection as they provide a way in for bugs. Anyone with a catheter needs to be aware that they are at risk of urine infections. Catheters can be used for both men and women, and though cumbersome shouldn't preclude you from intimacy. If you suffer from incontinence they can provide comfort and dryness, especially if you can't get out of bed.
- **What is a conveen?** This is a sheath that goes over the penis allowing urine to flow without leakage and so avoiding a catheter. It's another way of keeping dry when mobility is problematic.

- **What is a stoma?** A stoma is a part of the bowel that is brought out to the skin, during surgery, to allow the bowel contents or stool to pass into a collecting bag (stoma bag). The bag has an adhesive edge that sticks to the skin so that there is no leakage. This usually means no further stools are passed from the back passage, though there can still be some activity which varies from person to person. There are specialist stoma nurses who help with managing the bags, ensuring a good fit and correct size.
- **What is a PEG?** If eating is difficult, such as after a stroke or throat surgery, then a tube can be passed into the stomach through the skin of the stomach wall, to allow liquid feed to be given via a pump. It is called a PEG or a RIG. It is inserted in hospital, where the feed is also started. If you can manage your own pump then you will be shown how to use it during your hospital stay. Medication can also be given through this tube. If it falls out it can be reinserted but this has to be done in hospital. A PEG is different to a venting gastrostomy, which is also a tube in the stomach but this allows content out rather than in, so as to avoid vomiting when there is obstruction in the bowel, allowing patients to continue to eat.

There are more aids not mentioned here, a multitude to try to improve life for people with different problems. The best person to explain how to use and manage them is usually either the District Nurse or Clinical Nurse Specialist.

9. ACHES AND PAINS
SYMPTOM MANAGEMENT

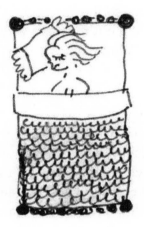

'I thought I'd get more pain. It's alright, I can manage. It wasn't like this with Janet, my wife. She really suffered. But then there wasn't all this help back then, was there?' **Alan, 77**

'Does it mean I can't drive? I've got to be able to drive. And look after the kids. Oh why did this have to happen?' **Ian, 49**

In this chapter we're going to focus on your continued physical care. We'll look at symptom management and the many ways we have of easing suffering. We've tried to be as comprehensive as space allows so you can find the answer you're looking for. However, reading about symptoms you *don't* have can cause unnecessary distress, so instead of reading the chapter from start to finish, we recommend you look for the symptom(s) you are experiencing to find out what is available to help you and leave it there.

9.1 Pain

'I didn't want Morphine but it's really worked. Frank takes me up to the club and I can do a bit on the golf course. Seeing friends is so important.' **Phoebe, 58**

Firstly, do note that **pain is NOT always a feature of a terminal illness**. Around 30% of cancer patients get no pain at all. People with other diseases can also have pain, and it's really important to let your medical team know so they can help. Pain is harder to assess in patients with dementia but there are ways of trying to measure this such as the Abbey Pain Scale.

9.1i Assessing pain

In order to help with pain, the team need to know what you're going through, as pain is invisible. It can't be physically measured; it can't be seen. We can hear it when someone shouts out, or recognise it when people grimace. How we each experience pain is incredibly varied.

Describing your pain will help your team understand how best to treat it. The features we look out for are:

- Where is it?
- Does it come and go or is it there all the time?
- Does it move? Go somewhere else? This is called 'radiation'.
- What does it feel like? Common sensations include aching, burning, stabbing, shooting.
- How disabling is it? What does it stop you doing?
- Does anything you've tried help to relieve it? Positional changes or heat pads can bring comfort.
- Does anything make it worse? Movement is often a trigger of arthritic pains.
- Is it there now?

If your pain comes and goes, it can be hard to remember, so writing down its features when you feel able may help the team better treat you. (You may like to use the space for notes in this paperback.) This is because different pains often require different medications or interventions.

'Pain scores' are commonly used, pain being measured on a scale of 1-10, where 1 is very little to 10 being unbearable. These scores can be hard to understand at first: I remember one patient shouting at the ward doctor, as he asked for his 'pain score' for the umpteenth time that day: *It's bloody 10!!!*' All he wanted was the Morphine, which was working well but not being given frequently enough. The point of the scoring is to better understand what you are feeling. What the teams need to know is how is the pain affecting you, what is it stopping you from doing and what have they tried that's done any good? This is why the questions above are worth answering, if you can, as they can be more helpful than a more generalised score.

Painkillers are known as 'analgesics' in the medical world. The advice from the World Health Organisation on treating pain is to start with the least medication needed and to climb 'the analgesic ladder' as required.

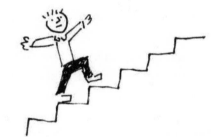

9.1ii Analgesics

Step 1: Paracetamol
Don't underestimate how effective this simple medication can be. Paracetamol can sometimes be enough to control your pain. It can work well with the opioids listed below, enhancing their effect. Paracetamol usually has few side effects and is well tolerated. If your liver is damaged the dose may be reduced.

Step 2: Weak opioids
These include Codeine and Tramadol. These work for the aches and deeper pains we can feel. They also help with colicky pains, headaches and sore joints. Common side effects include nausea (which should go after a few days), constipation, (which doesn't go and almost always requires laxatives), and drowsiness (which can be helpful at bedtime).

Step 3: Strong Opioids

Morphine is the best known strong opioid. It is cheap, available as tablets, liquid and injection, and highly effective in many severe pains. Side effects are similar to codeine: nausea, constipation and drowsiness. Other opioids work in slightly different ways, and are used in differing circumstances:

- Diamorphine is a close relative of Morphine and is easier to use if needing to give injections in higher doses.
- Oxycodone is synthetic opioid, i.e. made from chemicals and often used if you're allergic to Morphine or if your kidneys aren't working well.
- Fentanyl is another synthetic opioid that is usually applied to the skin in patch form every three days. Fentanyl patches are useful if there are difficulties swallowing tablets or absorbing medication through your bowel. Buprenorphine is another patch opioid, often used in osteoarthritic pain.
- There are also quick release versions of Fentanyl that can be given under the tongue, or melted in the cheek, giving swift relief, lasting usually up to an hour, lessening troublesome lingering side-effects. This can be particularly useful if your pain only occurs for brief times.

Other opioids include Pethidine, Hydromorphone, and Alfentanil, though these tend to be only used in special circumstances.

Fears about using drugs

Fear of using Morphine and related drugs is common. There are concerns around driving, sleepiness, addiction and hastening the end. Please be reassured that Morphine is a safe drug if used for pain in the dose required to keep it at a bearable level. Once the dose is stable, then you should be able to drive again. The sleepiness should pass after a few days. But if you

---

feel drowsy or unstable on your feet on this drug, then it's best to ask someone else to drive. Your doctor will be better placed to give more exact advice for your situation. If you are in bad pain and the Morphine-like drugs work, then it's unlikely you will get addicted. Addiction is a different disease, where drugs are used inappropriately for leisure or escape. If your pain improves, the doses are reduced and, as long as you don't stop them suddenly, you shouldn't notice any adverse effects.

Increasing use of pain-relieving medication can happen in the last few days of life, as sometimes the symptoms that have been a feature of the illness can worsen. This is appropriate and does not mean that the medication is reducing the time ahead. Instead it is keeping the patient pain-free and comfortable.

EXAMPLE 1

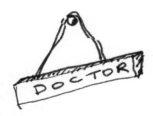

Suki has come to see Amina, the Consultant for a review of her pain.

'Suki, we last met a week ago. How have things been?'

'Not great. The pain has been less often but I feel so sleepy! I feel like I'm losing days.'

'OK, we'll look at that. Anything else going on?'

'I'm really down again. My last scan showed the disease has spread and I haven't told Aki. I can't bear to.'

'Was he not with you at the hospital?'

'No, he had to stay home to look after the kids. My mum was supposed to come but she had a cold.'

'I'm really sorry to hear that. Shall we talk about the scan?'

'No, they went through it all. I'm seeing Jackie next, the counsellor. I'll talk to her if you don't mind. I can't keep talking about it!'

131

'Of course, I do understand. But if you want to talk about things let me know. Let's look at your medication. You're on Paracetamol four times a day, Gabapentin 300mg three times a day, and 40mg Morphine capsules twice a day. Do you need any of the extra liquid Morphine in between times'?

'No, I've not used it at all. Should I be taking it as well?'

'Only if you need it. It's there if you have a flare up of pain. It can take 20 to 30 minutes to work, but then it should last around 3-4 hours. What we could try today is reducing your 12-hour Morphine to 30mg twice daily, and see if you need any extra top-up liquid. I'll get Shana, your Macmillan nurse, to call in a few days and see how you're doing?'

'Yes, that sounds good. I'll try that.'

'Hopefully you'll feel less drowsy. Bowels working OK?'

'Yes, I'm taking that laxative stuff. It works!'

'Good! You need to keep on top of that. I'll do you a prescription for the Morphine and ask your GP to supply more. Have a word with Shana in the week and let's see if the changes help. Otherwise I'll see you in two weeks. Is that OK?'

'Thanks, Dr Amina. I really appreciate you coming here. I'll talk more next time.'

'OK, Suki. See you soon.'

Step 4: Adjuvants

Alongside opioids, we can also use medications called 'adjuvants' as they work in different ways to help alleviate pain. They can complement drugs like Paracetamol and Morphine.

9.1iii Non-steroidal Anti-Inflammatory Drugs (NSAIDs)

Ibuprofen and naproxen are the commonest of this type of drug. You'll most likely know ibuprofen as it can be bought at the chemist and is often used for headaches and the mild pains of everyday life. They are effective painkillers, in particular for joint pains and infected areas, but they are limited by their unhelpful and many side effects, which is why they carry a warning that they should not be used for any length of time. Unwanted potential effects include stomach bleeding, kidney injury and even, in rare cases, heart attacks. The common adage is: **use the lowest dose for the least amount of time.** But for some people, continuous use is needed, as for them the benefits outweigh the risks. Your doctor will help you decide if this is the right group of drugs for you. It is good practice to use another drug called a Proton Pump Inhibitor (PPI) at the same time, as this reduces the risk of bleeding. Common PPIs include Omeprazole and Lansoprazole.

9.1iv Steroids

For palliative care patients, the steroid Dexamethasone is commonly used. It works by reducing pressure from the swelling around cancers, by stimulating appetite and sometimes by reducing pain. Its use is important in the treatment of cancers affecting the spinal cord and brain, aiming to preserve function until other treatments such as radiotherapy can be given.

Prednisolone is a steroid used in lung disease and rheumatological diseases like rheumatoid arthritis. It can reduce wheeze caused by constricted airways and the complications of infection, and it can ease the pain of swollen joints.

At times steroids can seem like wonder drugs, creating feelings of wellbeing. However, their use is limited by their extensive side effects. They are stimulants and can make you feel much brighter, but for some people this leads to anxiety and sleeplessness. With prolonged use they can induce Type 2 diabetes or worsen pre-existing diabetes. They can thin bones, leading to potential fractures. They can cause weight gain, fluid retention and also weaken the muscles at the top of the legs making it difficult to stand up. It's a long list! But again it's a question of balancing positive effects with the negative. Steroids are ideally used for short periods of time to give maximum improvement and to minimise these potential harms. If you have concerns around using them please ask your team to discuss the pros and cons. You are likely to also be prescribed a PPI as above, to protect your stomach whilst on steroid medication.

9.1v Nerve pain or neuropathic pain agents

Damage to nerves can cause a certain kind of pain called 'neuropathic'. You may have had sciatica in the past. This is a common neuropathic pain that many of us have experienced – a searing low back pain that goes into the buttock and down the back of the leg. Neuropathic pain can occur anywhere in the body; it can come on after chemo and radiotherapy and surgery where it is a side effect of treatment, and it can occur by direct injury to the nerve from cancers, infection, or accident. It can also occur after bony injury when there is new pressure on a nerve due to a change in the local anatomy – for example after a hip or spinal bone fracture.

Neuropathic pain can be characterised as a burning or shooting pain, similar in nature to toothache – something we have all known. It can sometimes be described as gnawing or like a bolt of lightning. Neuropathic agents aim to downgrade the pain, reducing the signals that the nerves are sending. This group of drugs can work in very different ways.

- Amitriptyline is an old-fashioned antidepressant drug that in low doses can be very effective for these shooting, burning pains. It is also used to prevent migraines and for sciatica. Side effects include dry mouth, constipation and blurred vision. If you can tolerate it, chances are it will work. One of the benefits of Amitriptyline is that it is sedating, helping you to get a good night's sleep. And of course this is also its downside, as it can then cause morning grogginess.
- Gabapentin was created as an anti-epileptic drug but tends to be used mostly for pain now. It works on receptors in the spinal column, aiming to lessen the signals that tell the brain that you have pain. The dose is slowly increased over a few weeks until the pain is better controlled, or until side effects limit its use. It has a more expensive relative called Pregabalin, which is sometimes used if Gabapentin isn't tolerated, or if there are difficulties with the amount of tablets. Gabapentin is prescribed three to four times daily, whereas Pregabalin is usually effective twice daily.

- The remaining agents that can work on nerve pain are used second or third line as they tend to be less effective. These include the antidepressant Duloxetine, the local anaesthetic Lidocaine, the irritant chilli cream Capsaicin, and cooling Menthol cream. The creams seem to work by distracting the nerves to a new sensation, so that our brains don't pay as much attention to the pain we are experiencing. You may also hear about TENS machines[28], acupuncture and the wide array of alternative therapies out there for this disabling symptom.

> **If pain is problematic,** then the medical team will usually want to see you frequently to assess the benefits of the medication, and change them as appropriate. It is on-going work. Tablets and doses are tweaked to try to best suit you. Changing medication too quickly can be confusing, so we tend to advise no more than one change every 24 hours in an otherwise stable situation. Otherwise it's not clear what's working and what is causing harm.

TIP: If you are in pain ASK FOR HELP. DON'T WAIT! It may be that you have the right medication but aren't using it in the right way. It may be that the dose needs a simple adjustment. Most doctors know how to use these medications and you should be able to get advice 24 hours a day. Your local hospice should have a helpline number to give medication advice.

9.2 Sickness and loss of appetite

Enjoyment of food and drink is central to our wellbeing, as we explored in Chapter 6. We don't usually think about it, but the complexity of eating includes seeing and smelling food, feeling it and tasting it on our tongues, the satisfying swallow and the final pleasure of fullness. This can be all topsy-turvy in illness and can really upset our day-to-day pleasures.

Feeling sick is horrible and being sick is its evil companion. Alongside sickness, some patients lose their appetite completely. This can be a result of medication like chemotherapy or it can be a result of cancer itself, suppressing appetite directly. As with nausea, it's debilitating and interferes with normal life. Chewing food when you don't want to, or that tastes of nothing is unsatisfying.

As with pain, it's helpful, if not very nice, to talk through what your sickness and appetite feels like:

- How often is it happening? Is it constant or only related to food?
- Does anything make it better? Sometimes being sick relieves nausea. Sometimes shifting position in bed does the trick.
- Does anything make it worse? The smell of food can be a trigger for example.
- Has anything you've tried helped?
- Has it come on with a new medication? Ask your doctor if you feel your nausea may be from your medication.

Simple measures to relieve nausea include:

- Eating smaller amounts more often.
- Eating what you fancy, not what you think you need. A bowl of ice cream can feel like a victory, whereas a bacon sandwich can feel like it will clog up your dry mouth.
- Don't necessarily stick to mealtimes. Eat when you feel like it, even if you've only just had a bowl of soup an hour ago.
- Make sure you're not constipated as this will only makes matters worse.

Simple measures around loss of appetite include:

- Not forcing yourself to eat. This may only make you feel worse.
- Understanding from your loved ones that this isn't rejection of their lovely food and care. It is part of the disease and it's OK to leave you be.

- Eating when you can't face it is unlikely to alter how your disease is progressing.
- If there are times you do fancy something, have what you enjoy, in manageable portions.

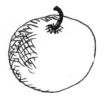 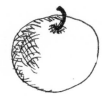 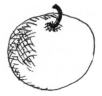

Common drugs that help nausea include Prochlorperazine (Stemetil), Cyclizine and Metoclopramide. They work in different ways, and your medical team will advise which is the most appropriate for your symptoms. There are lots of other drugs to help alleviate sickness, including Ondansetron, Haloperidol and Levomepromazine, all used for different indications. They work on different parts of your brain and bowel to help alleviate your symptoms. The choice of which one to use is often down to understanding the cause, and knowing potential side-effects, such as drowsiness or constipation.

Steroids like Dexamethasone can sometimes stimulate appetite. Taste should slowly return once chemotherapy has stopped – but frustratingly it doesn't always happen.

As with all medication, it's a balance of effect versus side effect. If you feel it is making things worse, please let your team know. They won't be able to guess and sometimes forget to ask directly.

9.3 Constipation and diarrhoea

Illness can present a dizzying array of horrible feelings. Feeling bunged up adds to nausea, makes you feel bloated and tired, and can cause pain. I didn't realise I would spend half my career talking about bowels, but ensuring a good motion gives such a feeling of wellness that we often take it for granted.

Medication, along with lack of activity, dehydration and general illness all contribute to constipation. The remedies vary according to what your poo is like: hard pellets, large dry stools or not going at all for days. And yes, as I talk about this all the time it causes me no embarrassment. We're trying to make you feel better. Laxatives, or aperients as they are also known, include:

- Softeners – to soften hard stools that are difficult to pass. These 'softeners' include Lactulose liquid, Docusate capsules and Movicol/Laxido sachets.
- Stimulants – to encourage the bowel to empty. These 'pushers' include Senna, Biscodyl, and Picosulfate.
- Usually a combination of softener and pusher is the best way forward e.g. Lactulose and Senna.
- Suppositories and enemas – if you haven't opened your bowels for a while pushing from the top doesn't always solve the problem. A little stimulation from below can do the trick. Glycerol and Bisacodyl suppositories or even Phosphate enemas can be used.

It's a case of getting the right combination in the right dose to get a more normal bowel movement. Spending time getting it right may be frustrating but once conquered it really does make a difference to how you feel.

The opposite symptom, diarrhoea, can be just as disabling: soiling without warning, a sore bottom from too frequent wiping and the worry of dehydration. The aim here is to reduce the bowel's activity without causing the constipated symptoms above.

- Reducing stimulant intake – avoid caffeine or eating spicy foods. Beans and pulses can also be highly propulsive!
- Loperamide (Imodium) – this opioid is the mainstay of slowing your bowel down. It utilises the constipating side effect of Morphine without being absorbed so you don't get the pain killer effects or the nausea. You can also buy this drug over the counter at the chemist.

- Codeine – as for Loperamide, this works as an opioid, but it is absorbed into the body and so provides pain relief too. It's a good choice if you have both pain and diarrhoea.

TIP: Be open and frank about your symptoms. The doctors and nurses are used to talking these things through and won't be upset by what you're telling them.

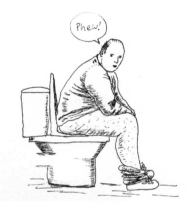

EXAMPLE 2

Suki meets up with her Macmillan nurse, Shana.

'*Hi Suki, how are you doing?*'

'*I'm more awake thanks, but I'm spending half my time trying to go to the loo and the other half trying to eat! I've lost some more weight. Aki keeps giving me large bowls of food, but I can't face it and he gets all upset.*'

'*OK, let's go through this in some detail. Are you feeling sick?*'

'*Not at all. I just have no appetite.*'

'*When you do eat, does the food have flavour?*'

'*No, it's like chewing cardboard. And tea tastes weird now.*'

'*Is swallowing alright?*'

'*Yes, it's fine. But everything is dry.*'

Shana has a look in Suki's mouth. Her tongue is furred up with oral thrush.

'*Looks like you have an infection on your tongue, Suki. This can make food tasteless and give you a dry mouth. I'll give you something to help that. Now let's look at your bowels. How often are you going to the loo?*'

'I'm trying to go! I get the urge, then nothing happens. It's been over a week now.'

'What are you taking for it?'

'I stopped taking the Senna as I was getting stomach ache. So I'm only taking Lactulose now. A spoon at night.'

'That's probably not enough.'

'But I don't want the runs!'

'Sure, I understand. I think the stomach ache may be more likely to be from the constipation itself. Let's restart the Senna and increase the Lactulose to two spoonfuls twice a day. With the Senna you can take two at night if you haven't been, or only one if you have. That way you shouldn't get the runs!'

Suki laughs. 'I'd be glad of something happening down there. I feel so bloated!'

'Let's try that. Is Aki here?'

'He's at work.'

'I'll leave you both a leaflet about diet. But Suki, it's fine to eat what *you* want. If Aki is giving you too much, it's probably because he wants to help. It's worth letting him know that it's the disease that is stopping you eating. It's not your choice. It can be really hard for him to understand when he's trying to be there for you.'

'Hmph! It's harder for me! But I take your point.'

'Let's make sure that next time I come back that you're both here, then if it's still an issue, we can look at this together.'

9.4 Breathlessness

We've all felt breathless after running or exercising vigorously, but if this is how you feel just walking from one room into another, it can be very distressing. Managing breathlessness is a combined effort of looking at your lung and heart function, assessing medication, checking your oxygen levels when you move, and trying to formulate a regimen that will work for you individually.

Lung disease springs to mind when we think about breathlessness, but it can also happen in any cancer due to anaemia or weight loss, in heart failure when the heart isn't pumping properly, and in neurological disorders when the nerves don't move the breathing muscles well enough to provide the exchange of carbon dioxide waste for the refreshment of oxygen.

There are a few ways to manage this disabling sensation. Occupational and physiotherapists are excellent at helping and may suggest:

- **Knowing your limits.** Take regular rests when moving so as to catch your breath. Do this more often if you're very breathless. Perhaps organise seating on your regular routes around the house – a perching stool placed in the hall, a barstool in the kitchen for cooking, a chair in the bathroom to have a rest after you get out of the shower or bath.
- **Getting fresh air.** Keeping windows open and using electric fans can give the sensation that breathing is easier. Have a fan by you, in your hand, at your bedside and when you are going out. It's like having the car window open, giving a feeling of freshness. Some like a constant flow, others prefer the swinging fan as it tilts from side to side. I've seen breathless patients feeling quite settled, wearing big duvets to keep warm whilst a cold fan is blasting on their face.
- **Practising breathing techniques** – breathlessness can feel frightening. Patients report feelings of panic frequently. They are shown that their oxygen level is normal but still they breathe fast and in an uneven way, exacerbating the sensation. Learning to slow your breathing down can help to remedy matters. The common advice is to 'breathe around a rectangular window'.
  - Take a breath in as you SLOWLY follow the short side of the window with your eyes, breathe out MORE SLOWLY as your eyes travel along the longer side of the window, then breathe in again on the third short side, and then out MORE SLOWLY on the final fourth longer panel.
  - Slowing the rate down can feel like the wrong thing to do as there is a strong desire to breathe more quickly, but with training you can gain better control.

141

Another technique is *the calm hand* illustrated here, which follows similar principles:

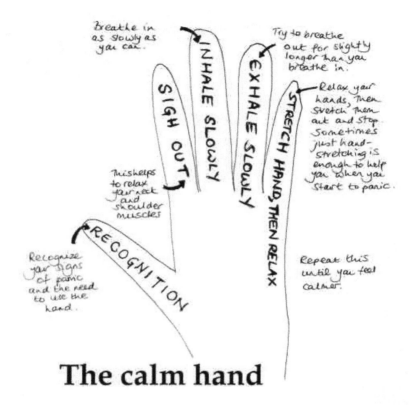

Breathe in as slowly as you can.

Try to breathe out for slightly longer than you breathe in.

Relax your hands, then stretch them out and stop. Sometimes just hand-stretching is enough to help you when you start to panic.

INHALE SLOWLY

EXHALE SLOWLY

SIGH OUT

STRETCH HAND, THEN RELAX

This helps to relax your neck and shoulder muscles

RECOGNITION

Recognize your signs of panic and the need to use the hand.

Repeat this until you feel calmer.

The calm hand

- If your breathlessness is causing great anxiety and worry, then using a calming medication like Lorazepam can help to soothe these feelings. A bit like a pint of beer.
- Morphine can be an aid to breathlessness too. It tells the brain's respiratory centre to calm down a little, to take your time, to breathe a little slower.
- Paradoxically, oxygen doesn't always satisfy the feelings of breathlessness. This is often because blood oxygen levels don't match the sensation of breathlessness. Referral to a respiratory nurse can help clarify its use: they will measure blood oxygen levels and see if it is low at rest, on movement, or normal. Often levels are normal despite feeling that they

are low, so extra oxygen is of limited use. Exceptions of course exist, and these include patients with pulmonary fibrosis, who may benefit from higher doses of oxygen, and some COPD and heart failure patients, who may only require a tiny amount, say one to two litres, to feel better.

- Non-invasive ventilation (NIV). In some circumstances our lungs need more help. NIV is a type of machine that pushes air into the lungs enabling breathing to be less laboured. Patients with some kinds of COPD and MND benefit greatly from this treatment. A mask is applied tightly to the face and air, with or without extra oxygen, is pushed firmly but gently into the lungs. The down side is that the mask is tight on the face and the machine is noisy. Wearing a mask limits talking and eating too. The up side is that it can reduce the effort of breathing. Once used to it, many patients report great benefit.

9.5 Skin Health

Longer illnesses can threaten the skin's normal barrier, allowing infection or sores to develop. Here are a few issues that may arise:

- Medication can cause rashes.
- Skin can dry out and get cracked, leading to local infection.
- Resting for too long on one area can reduce the oxygen flow, leading eventually to break down of the skin and ulceration.
- Irritant reactions in the groin can occur following prolonged exposure to urine or faeces in people who have incontinence.

If you notice any changes to your skin do let the teams know. Examination will help them better understand what's causing it and what the treatment might be.

- People staying mostly in bed need to have their skin checked on a daily basis to ensure that problem areas are given relief, by regular turning and use of pressure-relieving mattresses. Frequent checks and changes, along with barrier creams and sprays can help reduce problems.

Another issue that may arise is swelling, as some illnesses interrupt the flow of lymph fluid. This is a watery substance that seeps naturally from the blood stream into the surrounding tissue where it is picked up again by the lymph drainage system. Blockages at any point can mean holding of the fluid within the skin, leading to swelling. This is called lymphoedema. It can happen after lymph node surgery following breast cancer treatment and also in heart failure where swollen lower legs get very sore and wet. Alongside the District Nurses, there are specialist nurses at the hospice who can help with easing the swelling with massage, pressure stockings and skin moisturisers.

TIP: If you develop unexpected swelling in your lower leg, there is a possibility that a clot has formed in a vein (Deep Vein Thrombosis or DVT). The swelling is at the back, in the calf muscles, and can also be sore and red, but isn't always. Cancer, recent surgery, and reduced mobility all increase chances of a DVT. The worry is that it can break off, pass up the vein to the lungs where it can lodge, preventing normal function. This is called a Pulmonary Embolus (P.E.). If the clot is big enough this can be fatal. Always show any leg swelling to your doctor as soon as you find it – they are best placed to diagnose a cause. Don't wait: if your GP surgery is shut, attend Out Of Hours or A&E – this is a potential emergency.

Blood thinners are used to either prevent this from happening or to treat it if it has happened. These include injections into the stomach skin with a version of a drug called Heparin – common names include Dalteparin and Tinzaparin – or tablet form, which includes Warfarin, Apixiban and Rivaroxiban. The choice and dose of blood thinner will depend on your individual circumstances.

9.6 Further complications

As you might imagine, there are as many unexpected complications possible as diseases that exist. The likelihood of these happening will depend on the illness and how it is progressing. DVT is one of the commoner occurrences but on the whole these are rare.

The following is only for information and not to scare you. It may be beneficial to know that bad things can happen, as if you spot them early you can be ready. For example:

- Cancers tend to have lots of blood vessels within them. Very rarely these can become unstable and bleeding occurs. If you see any bleeding – in your spit, stool, urine, skin – let your team know. Remedies are various and include radiotherapy, cautery and medication to stem the flow.
- Infections can also increase with illness. This is often the case in lung disease where the ability of the lung to clean itself is reduced. COPD is characterised by having repeated infections. It may be useful to have antibiotics at home if you're getting repeated infections so that you can start treatment early. Urine infections are commoner in those who have a catheter and those whose immune system is suppressed, such as following chemotherapy.
- Symptoms of infection can be fever, increased pain, shivers and shakes, and vomiting.
- Other complications we have discussed already include spinal cord compression, where cancer has spread to the spinal bones and is pushing on the cord, causing pain and loss of function (see page 113). Increasing confusion can occur quickly, for example due to excess medication, infection, or chemical imbalance like rising calcium levels.
- Severe chest pain can be linked to a heart attack, and signs of a drooping face with limb weakness can be suggestive of a stroke happening. **Act quickly, dial 999.**

TIP: This list of physical symptoms isn't exhaustive. I've only mentioned the common symptoms people can feel. Don't let this stop you mentioning something we haven't talked about here, as something you feel may be trivial may be of concern to your doctor. For example, increasing breathlessness may be part of your disease process, but it may also mean something else is happening which is potentially treatable e.g. anaemia, which can be treated with a blood transfusion.

We're nearly through with this chapter. But before we go, let's catch up with Suki one more time.

EXAMPLE 3

Suki and Aki meet up at the hospice with Shana and Dr Amina.

'Hi there,' says Dr Amina. 'I'm glad we could all get together today. Thank you for coming in. How are things going?'

'They're not' says Suki.

'And for you, Aki?'

'It's getting harder. Suki isn't eating anything now. She just lies down all the time. I have to do everything, which is fine, but I'm tired and worried.'

'What do you think, Suki?'

'He's right. I'm spending most of the time on the sofa. I want so much to be with everyone but it tires me out. I just sleep.'

'How are you physically, are your symptoms OK?' asks Shana.

'No, my pain is bad again, and at the same time I'm exhausted. The constipation is better but I still don't want to eat.'

'Sounds like a lot is going on, Suki,' says Amina. 'Have you any thoughts as to how we could help today?'

There is silence for a moment.

'It's OK to talk about anything,' Amina says quietly.

'I feel a burden,' says Suki.

'You're not a burden! What are you saying?' Aki says.

'It's how I feel. I wish I could do more. I wish this would stop.'

Aki and Suki both look at the floor, tearful.

'Perhaps one thing we could look at is a little time at the hospice,' suggests Amina.

146

'What, to die?' asks Suki.

'I don't think you're at that stage yet, Suki. But if things change more quickly then, yes, you can stay at the hospice if that feels appropriate. I was thinking more along the lines of coming in for a couple of weeks to assess your symptoms and treat them more fully, giving Aki and yourself some time away from the worries of home. Then returning home feeling a little better.'

There is more quietness as this offer is digested.

'Is she dying?'

'Not today, Aki, but things are changing, aren't they? We're seeing more time resting, less eating, more weariness and fatigue. It all suggests that the disease is progressing.'

'Can I think about it?' asks Suki.

'Of course,' says Shana. 'I'll find out if there is a bed. Perhaps when the next one comes available we can talk about it?'

'I think I'd like that,' says Suki.

I appreciate this chapter is a difficult read. If you're struggling, now might be a good time to re-read Chapter 7, and seek support from some of the people we discussed there.

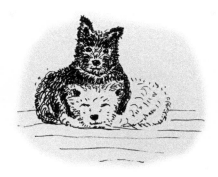

For your own notes:

....

....

....

....

....

....

....

....

....

....

....

....

....

....

....

....

V. PLANNING FOR THE FUTURE

10. THE LAW

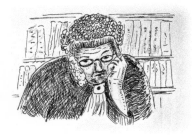

'I wish he had left a will. I wouldn't be in this mess.' **Doreen, 88**

'I really don't want to go back to hospital. EVER AGAIN! I don't want to be poked, given tubes of stuff, bloody leave me alone.' **Phil, 77**

In the midst of illness it can seem impossible to think clearly about the future. There's so much going on – seeing doctors, explaining to family and friends what is happening to you. Advice flies around and it can be bewildering: you should do this, you should do that. As well-meaning as everyone is, this can be a lot to take in, especially when you're trying to cope with your condition.

TIP: And now here I come with some more advice! One thing that can make it a little easier is to think about your wishes and hopes for the future and to write these down. If there are things you DON'T want to happen to you, then there are processes to make your decisions formal and legal. You can change your mind at any point but it gives the people around you strong guidance as to what matters to you.

If the following information appears to be written in a more formal manner, this is because it needs to be as exact as possible, and the law tends to be cut and dried. We've tried to make this book as clear, comprehensive and gentle as possible, and aim to do that here, too. Sometimes, however, the law can be like a thorny maze: you may think you have found the way forward, only to get caught on another barb. Bear with us and we'll try our best try to guide you through.

10.1 Making a will

If you want to leave different things to different people, then *please write a will.* I recommend most people do this as soon as possible, even if they are in excellent health. It makes certain what will happen to your home and belongings, from large items like cars and houses, to small personal mementos which make a strong tie between you and a loved one. If you are married and have no will, then your belongings will pass to your spouse – this is cheaper and easier if that is all you want to do. Also, if your family get on and you can be confident that they won't argue about who gets what then you, too, should be able to get away without a will.

Dying without a will is called 'being intestate' and means that the government can take control of your estate. **They will organise for it to be given to your immediate family but not to your partner unless you are legally married or in a civil partnership.** There is detailed information from the government which you can access online at gov.uk/inherits-someone-dies-without-will but **a will is easy to write and you don't always have to have a lawyer.**

TIP: There are packs to help you write a will available in high street shops and online. A lawyer can help in more complicated situations if you are leaving lots of different items or money to quite a few people or setting up trusts, and in some circumstances this may give you added peace of mind. If you are worried about the expense of a lawyer, there may be a social worker at the hospice who can give guidance.

When writing a will, remember it needs to be clear, definite, then dated and witnessed to make it legal. Advice on how to write wills can be found at the government website[29] and also at independent sites such as Money Advice[30].

10.2 Capacity and the Mental Capacity Act

Whilst you are well and able to communicate your decisions, then your opinion is paramount, and you are deemed to have capacity. This means that if you are offered a treatment, then you get to decide if you want it or not. A trickier situation arises when you are not able to communicate your wishes or if you appear confused. This can be due to a number of causes. Although mental capacity issues commonly arise in advanced dementia, they are not confined to this condition. I have seen people struggle with capacity and decision-making due to brain tumours, to advanced disease where are they too frail to communicate, and due to accident or head injury.

We can live any way we chose – in a tent, dressed as a gorilla, up a tree – providing we can pay for it, it's legal, and the decision is our own to make.

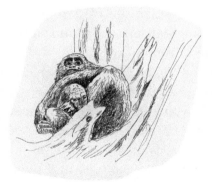

If we become unable to make decisions, or we are unable to communicate any decisions, then the Mental Capacity Act (MCA) can be invoked. If the medical team feel that you are unable to make a decision about your care, and a decision needs to be made, then they need to consider invoking the MCA. The MCA says that certain tests are done to see if someone lacks the capacity to make a decision. Prior to testing, capacity must be assumed to exist. Testing can be done by doctors, mental health teams and social workers.

The tests are two-fold. Firstly, the Act asks, does the person have a condition interfering with their normal brain functioning? If so, does it interfere to the point of affecting decision-making? If the answer is 'yes', then they proceed to the next questions:

- Can the person understand the information they are being given?
- Can they keep this information in their minds over a period of time?
- Can they weigh up the implications of the information they are being given?
- Can they communicate their decision?

If the answers to ANY of the four questions above is 'No', then the person is deemed likely to lack the capacity to make a decision pertaining to their health and/or finances.

Professionals are obliged to make it as easy as possible for the person to understand the information. So questions need to be offered by any appropriate means of communication – for example via a translator, or using sign language, loud volume or touch. Talking isn't the only way to communicate.

The onus is also on the professional to ensure the questions are asked in a way that gives the person the best chance of answering. An extreme example would be someone who can't speak or use hand gestures. The professional could ask about the person's preferences using questions that can be answered 'yes' or 'no', and the person could be asked to blink once for 'yes' and twice for 'no'. You can imagine how difficult it can be to ascertain all of this, and how it can potentially be open to abuse. Delirium in hospital is common. Someone may have an infection that causes confusion, but when treated, they are clear in their thinking again. The Act asks of professionals:, does this decision need to be made now? Can it wait until an opportunity that the patient has regained capacity?[31]

If there is conflict around decisions for someone lacking capacity, then the team can organise a Best Interests meeting. This is a gathering of everyone involved in a patient's care, from health professionals to carers to loved ones, where the aim is to reach an agreement as to the best way forward at that time[32].

EXAMPLE 1

We met Dora earlier, in Chapter 5; she is our older woman, with dementia. Now Dora has a chest infection. Her two sons, John and Tony, both have strong ideas around her future care. Let's meet them at her care home in discussion with Dr Ahmed, GP.

'Mum has to go to hospital,' says John, the older son. 'The antibiotics aren't working, are they?

'Her infection hasn't responded to them in the way I had hoped,' says Dr Ahmed.

'Then she needs to be treated,' says John.

'What do you think, Tony?' asks Dr Ahmed.

'She looks really comfortable here. What would we achieve by sending her to hospital, when she's only going to get another infection when she comes back? It's like a merry-go-round.'

'What do you think your mum would have wanted?'

John frowns. 'Mum always said, "I don't want to be in a care home." Yet here she is. She'd hate this.'

'She would hate it.' Tony nods. 'But she isn't aware, is she? And we need to help her as best as we can.'

'Your mum can't decide what to do next, so we have to do that on her behalf,' says Dr Ahmed. 'She has had three infections in the past few months, each needing a hospital admission. Afterwards she has come home, looking frailer, and now she is spending all of her time in bed. She has lost a lot of weight. All of this tells me that her dementia has progressed and that time ahead is short. I also know that if we don't admit her she may die of this infection.'

'Admit her then,' says John.

'Hasn't she had enough?' asks Tony. 'What do you think, doctor?'

'I think these decisions are really hard to make. From what you tell me, *your mother would not like to be in the condition that she is in now. I don't think any of us would. I also know from experience that she may die from this infection, but that may happen in hospital too.'*

'Oh, I don't want that!' says John.

'Me neither.'

'OK. We could try switching her to a different antibiotic and see how she goes,' says Dr Ahmed. 'Then we could meet up again in a couple of days to see how things are.'

'No, just leave her be,' says Tony. 'No more tablets.'

'John?' asks Dr Ahmed.

'If it's as bad as you say, let's keep Mum comfortable here. I don't want her being jostled around, lying on a trolley for hours. God, it's horrible.'

'It's really hard,' says Dr Ahmed. 'Let's get the staff to come in and we'll let them know our decision to keep your mother here. I can also let the ambulance and our Out-of-Hours services know, in case they get involved. Then everyone is aware what we have decided.'

Tony and John agree.

Dora doesn't get better. Gradually, over the next few days, she becomes more and more sleepy. She dies peacefully a few days later with her sons at her bedside.

TIP: One way to help in these difficult situations is to grant someone you know and trust the ability to make decisions on your behalf, should you become incapacitated. This is known as Lasting Power of Attorney. Another way is to make your decisions NOT to have treatment known in advance, known as Advance Decisions to Refuse Treatment (ADRT).

10.3 Lasting Power of Attorney (LPA)

Lasting Power of Attorney means that you can give control of your decisions to someone close to you, someone you trust, who knows your mind well. If you are no longer able to decide, then they can decide on your behalf.

There are two kinds of LPA – one for finance and one for health. That means that there are **two** forms to fill in and to pay for. People often organise this at the same time as doing their wills. Let's take a look at the differences.

10.3i LPA for Property and Finance

This LPA is to ensure that your finances can be organised by someone else if you are unable to make decisions. It is the commoner used of the two, as often we rely on medical teams to make decisions around health. Should you lose capacity, your nominated Attorney – the person who you have entrusted to make decisions on your behalf – will be able to access your bank accounts, thereby getting your bills paid, paying for services like carers, and being able to use your money to buy you clothes and food. If you need to live in a care home – residential or nursing – then they can sell your property to pay for this.

> **FACT: If you don't have an LPA, it will be down to your Local Authority to make these decisions. But don't worry – nothing can happen whilst you can make and communicate decisions, this only applies if you no longer have that ability.**

You can make your own LPA online at the Government website here: www.gov.uk/power-of-attorney/overview and www.gov.uk/lasting-power-attorney-duties/property-financial-affairs. **Doing this yourself online is cheaper than getting a lawyer to do it** but if your property and finances are complicated it may be wise to get professional legal advice.

If you don't have an LPA and lose capacity, your family will be consulted around decisions by the Local Authority, but they won't have final say. Ideally, everyone is in agreement, so this isn't an issue. However, if there are concerns and your loved ones want to be in control of your finances, they would need to apply to the Court of Protection in order to access your estate. This is often costly but it is doable and gives you the equivalent of an LPA. It can be cheaper to do this online but you may prefer to use a solicitor.

If you no longer have capacity and have no family or LPA, then the Local Authority will provide an IMCA (independent mental capacity advocate) to ensure that decisions around your care are being made in your best interests[33].

10.3ii LPA for Health

In the UK, decisions around health are decided by doctors if the patient is unable to contribute to that decision. Families will be consulted for their opinion, but doctors have the final say on which treatments to offer and which to withhold. As a patient, you are usually deeply involved in these decisions.

Imagine if you could not be involved though, if, say, you had a heart attack or a stroke? **It may be important to you NOT to have certain treatments. Your Attorney for Health – the person you nominate via your LPA – will be able to make these decisions on your behalf.** Decisions can include difficult ethical issues, such as whether or not to treat you on the Intensive Care Unit, where machines will breathe for you, whether or not to use artificial feeding, or whether or not to try to restart your heart if it stops beating. If your wishes are already known to someone close to you, then they may be easier to make, but don't forget they can also be tricky for your LPA to manage when faced with complex situations. Instead, you may prefer to rely on your medical team to make these decisions for you. You can create your LPA form online[34] or via your solicitor.

10.4 Advance Decision to Refuse Treatment (ADRT)

As you can see, being prepared for unexpected events gives you more control over your life and belongings. An additional way to do this, along with the LPA documents above, is to **make written and witnessed decisions about your future care. This is called an**

Advance Decision To Refuse Treatment or ADRT[35]. You may know it from its previous name of Living Will.

Why is this important? If you are suffering from a progressive illness like dementia or motor neurone disease, you may not want certain interventions. For example, if you have difficulty swallowing, you may not want to be fed artificially, even though this could improve your quality of life. Inserting a tube into the stomach (PEG or RIG) means that food, fluids and medication can be given providing sustenance and relieving thirst and hunger. But if you are in a position where feeding will not change your prognosis, or if you are adamant you don't want this to happen, then an ADRT may be appropriate.

CPR, or cardiopulmonary resuscitation, is another procedure that you may not want. This is what you see on television, when a team of health professional are trying to restart the heart by pumping on the chest and breathing into the mouth. This procedure has a low success rate, and even lower if you have a life-shortening illness. If you don't want this to happen, you can make an ADRT to ensure it doesn't.

ADRTs need to be specific, e.g. *I do not want CPR under any circumstances; I do not want to be admitted to Intensive Care under any circumstances.* They also need to show that you understand the consequences and gravity of your decision: *I do not want to be artificially ventilated under any circumstances even if this results in my death.*

FACT: Health professionals will usually try to save your life if there is no documentation around.

ADRTs only work if they are known about by those involved in your care. Keep yours with you, and give a copy to your loved ones or make it available to those making decisions on your behalf. You can also think about keeping a copy in your District Nursing notes at home and make sure that your GP has a copy, as well as the local ambulance service and A&E department.

The problem with both LPA for Health and ADRTs is that circumstances can change, and situations that seemed so clear early on may be less clear when something happens. For instance, if you have an ADRT saying you don't want to be admitted to Intensive Care, what happens if all you need is 24 hours there and then you could be stepped down to a normal ward? They often involve difficult decisions to make in advance unless you have a very clear idea of the outcome. Though your doctor can't write the ADRT with you, they may be able to talk to you about the consequences.

> **FACT: It's important to note at this point that, in the UK, you can't demand a treatment. If the doctor feels the treatment is not useful they are not obliged to give it to you.**

TIP: This can occasionally lead to friction between patient and doctor, so getting the team to explain why an intervention might not be useful, won't work or isn't appropriate for you can help to lessen the fears that something is being missed.

Whilst you're in the process of making all these decisions around the future, why not **look back at the Advance Care Planning we discussed at the end of Chapter 2?** This is a statement of things that are important to you, such as where you would like to be cared for in the future, and also what you might hope to do with the time that lies ahead. You may decide this is all you can contemplate and, if so, that is OK. Just make a will and an Advance Care Plan or Statement, and leave it there. There are laws in place to look after you without an ADRT.

10.5 Do Not Attempt Cardiopulmonary Resuscitation (DNACPR)

The world of medicine is full of acronyms, which seem clear to the medical profession, but can be confusing to everyone else and here is a good example. **DNACPR or uDNACPR is a document** completed by a health professional, usually the most senior doctor, advising that attempts to try to restart the heart will NOT be made, if it stops beating. In simpler language, the teams won't try to restart the heart by pushing up and down on the chest. **This means that the patient is allowed to die a natural death.** For most people with life-limiting illnesses this seems to make sense, as trying to restart the heart is very likely not going to work. If it was successful, and the chances of this are remote, then the patient is brought back to die of their illness in a different way a little later. The heart stopping is the worst prognostic sign – it indicates very clearly that time ahead is extremely limited.

Confusion arises, I think, with the word 'resuscitation'. DNACPR only applies to the heart stopping. Patients can still have appropriate treatment at home or be admitted to hospital, for example to treat infections by intravenous antibiotics or fix broken bones. It doesn't mean you are abandoned. However, in our attempts at kindness at the end of life, it can seem like another hope is taken away.

For many patients this can be a straightforward decision, as they often say things like:

'I don't want anyone jumping up and down on my chest. What's the point?' **Wayne, 88**

On the other hand, some patients are desperate to try anything, including CPR. I had a patient willing to have CPR even though she had advanced cancer and heart failure and kidney failure:

'What else is there but another day to live?' **Prue, 99,** asked me, as though I was very stupid.

Though I explained that the attempt would likely be futile, and may cause distress, she was adamant. Despite the explanation of potentially fractured ribs, a trip to A&E and strangers pumping on her chest, this is what she wanted and whilst patients can't demand treatment, they also need our respect. I left the form uncompleted. In the end she died peacefully at home, her husband forgetting to call the ambulance. In this situation we see that avoiding CPR led to a peaceful, dignified death with Prue's husband present.

Here is a cold statistic about the success rates of CPR – it may help you better understand why these decisions are made.

Resuscitation council: *'In the UK fewer than 10% of all the people in whom a resuscitation attempt is made outside hospital survive.'*

You can read more at www.resus.org.uk/faqs/faqs-cpr/

Remember these statistics mostly include people who don't have a life-limiting illness. The General Medical Council's ethical stance on this issue is fairly extensive and can be read on their website[36].

TIP: The following section is quite dry I'm afraid, but it's important too. You may need to know where you stand in terms of work, sick leave and benefits. I can imagine reading this is like wading through glue, so perhaps skip to the bit you need now.

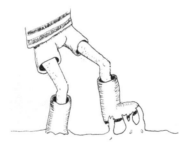

10.6 Work and the law

Just because you have a life-limiting illness doesn't mean you can't or shouldn't work, as we explored in Chapter 7. You may find it keeps you going, and that it is crucial to who you are as a person. However, if your disease if disabling, or you need time out of work for treatment, it's worth knowing what the law states. The gist is that if you can work, then it may be better to continue. If you don't feel up to it you can claim sick leave. If you don't have insurance to cover this, then you may need a 'Fit Note' from your GP.

If you feel able to, then talking to your employer is usually very helpful. Let your manager know what is happening to you, what time off you may need for treatment, and when you might be back. You can also ask them to keep this information to themselves and be discrete. Your employer needs to plan around your absence of leave, so the more notice you can give the better. If the company you work for is large enough, they may have an Occupational Health department. Discussions with them should help you find a way forward.

Discuss how much time you may need early on. For some jobs, it is seen as a bad thing if you have repeated episodes off work. Employers can get annoyed if you come and go with the same illness. **It may be better, though feel odd, to get a sick note for the whole time you need, particularly if this is around treatment.**

People with cancer are protected under the Disability Discrimination Act 1995. There is a guide available from Macmillan Cancer Care to help you with your employment rights. What it says is that you can't lose your job because of your illness. However, your employer may have some justification for removing you from employment if you are physically no longer able to do your job. They should try to accommodate you elsewhere, perhaps on different or lighter duties, but they are not always obliged and this can get really tricky as it will also depend on your job contract. Getting advice from your line manager, from your union, or from Citizens Advice may be worthwhile.

TIP: Try to get an agreement with your employer sorted early on.

Similar levels of protection are there for people with other life-limiting conditions. If you feel you are being discriminated against due to your illness, then please get in touch with your union representative. If you have no union, then please join one. If there is no obvious union for your job then you can find the right one for you at the TUC website[37].

10.6i Fit notes (formerly sick notes)

GPs can issue Fit Notes to give you time off work for ill health. The Fit Note gives two options. The first is to completely stop you working. This then entitles you to statutory sick pay if you earn over £112 a week. Otherwise you need to claim ESA (Employment Support Allowance) via the Job Centre. You can negotiate the length of time needed with your GP according to your circumstances. In the first instance, this is usually for two weeks, so that you can meet up again and see how things are going. Longer time off work can be given if needed. Sometimes you'll want time off to travel to and from treatment. Sometimes you may need a week off because you feel unwell and your symptoms are not controlled. And sometimes you need it because things are changing quickly and a return to work is not feasible.

The second type of Fit Note explains that you 'may be able to work' if work can be adapted to the changes you are experiencing. This can mean a change in hours, altered duties, adjusted workspace, or whatever it is that will keep things going. Employers are not obliged to follow the doctor's guidance but the note should give you a good degree of support.

The legal side of Fit Notes is covered on the Government website[38].

10.6ii Self-employment

Many people work for themselves. If you're self-employed and you stop working, then you have no income. If you are in this situation you may have bought insurance to cover eventualities like this, often called an Income Protection Plan. Now may be the time to cash this in. A financial advisor may be able to help with this. If you don't have a cushion of savings or insurance policy, please ensure that you have applied for the benefits listed below.

Whatever your disease, it's worth looking at this excellent page from Macmillan Cancer Support aimed at those who are self-employed. It gives advice on the pros and cons of being self-employed, flexibility versus lack of colleague support, and reiterates the need to check that you have all the benefits to which you are entitled[39].

Unfortunately getting grants and other financial help isn't easy or common.

TIP: If you have a mortgage, you may be able to get some leeway on your repayments. Speak to your mortgage lender as soon as you can.

10.6iii Dismissal

Employers are obliged to abide by the law. If you have a disability, then you are covered by the Disability Discrimination Act, which states that you cannot be dismissed due to a disability. However, if you are no longer able to do your job due to a change in your physicality then this becomes more problematic. I would again advise seeking guidance from Citizens Advice or from your solicitor.

If you feel you have been unfairly treated due to your illness you may also have rights to recompense. There is guidance from the government[40] urging employers to do all they can to accommodate change and ill health. You may need more detailed guidance, and the Equality Advisory Service[41] can help.

10.7 Debt

What a time to think about money! The stress of money never goes away, not in life, not during our last illness, not even after we have died. Sadly, there is nothing in the law protecting someone with a life-limiting illness from their debt responsibilities. Life insurance may cover some eventualities but the onus is on the person's estate to cover debts. Once the person has died, their estate pays the bills. Any benefactors are obliged to pay off debts from the estate but not from their own resources.

FACT: Your offspring won't be paying off your credit card bill or mortgage but they will only inherit what is left of your estate once bills have been deducted.

If you're struggling with debt, there are three very useful points of contact:

- **National Debtline:** 0808 808 4000
  www.nationaldebltline.org
- **Step Change Debt Charity:** 0800 138 1111
  www.stepchange.org
- **Debt Advice Foundation:** 0800 622 6151
  debtadvicefoundation.org

There is further guidance about debt and ill health at the Money Advice Service website[42].

Mortgages can be an issue if you have joint home ownership, as can joint accounts and joint investments. There is clear advice again from the Money Advice Service[43]. They also have a page[44] where you can get debt advice if you are in difficulties.

10.8 Gifts of money

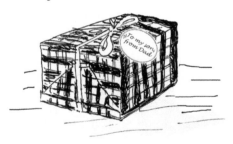

Would it be wise to transfer money from a joint account into your loved one's account so that this is no longer in your name? You may be thinking this in order to avoid paying duties to the government. There is difficulty here, as the Inland Revenue are aware of quick changes to accounts. You will definitely need advice from someone who knows about money, usually a lawyer, about the time frame around changing account names, mortgage names and moving money to a family member. Top line: we would advise you to be cautious.

10.9 Benefits to which you may be entitled

Having a serious illness entitles you to some benefits. We looked at some of these in Chapter 5, but I'd hate for you to miss out on your entitlements, so let's run through them again:

- **Attendance Allowance – for those over 65.** You can apply for Attendance Allowance if you are not able to look after yourself without help. It is paid at two different rates according to disability and not according to income. Details are on the government website[45].
- **Personal Independence Payments (PIPs) – for those under 65**. You will be entitled to PIP payments if you have a life-shortening illness and are under 65. It is calculated according to need and there is great advice on how to apply for it, as well as eligibility, on the Citizens Advice website[46]. Your GP will need to complete a form known as a DS1500 to send to Social Services. A DS1500 is completed if your health team feel it is likely that you have less than six months to live. These are hard emotive decisions, I do understand, but **you are entitled to the money regardless of income and it may come in handy.** And as we have seen, knowing how much time lies ahead is not an accurate science but an educated guess that things are changing enough to warrant completing this form.

TIP: To check what benefits you may be entitled to, try using the Citizens Advice Web Calculator.

10.10 Other grants

There may also be grants available for specific items if you are not able to afford them. These can include motorised wheelchairs and stair lifts – even respite care so that your carer can have a break. Once again, the charity websites are a good place to start. Here are some examples:

- www.mariecurie.org.uk/help/benefits-entitlements/getting-help/grants
- www.macmillan.org.uk/information-and-support/organising/benefits-and-financial-support/benefits-and-your-rights/macmillan-grants.html
- www.mndassociation.org/getting-support/financial-support-information-for-people-with-mnd/

…and you'll find more details at the end of this book.

There is also Continuing Health Care funding to consider, as discussed in Chapter 5.

TIP: The general advice with financial matters is to seek help early – don't wait until things mount up or get too difficult to untangle.

As you can see the law provides ways for you to plan your affairs, to have your say if you aren't able to speak for yourself, and to help with financial matters around work, debt and benefits. Though it can appear confusing and at times complex, it's there to protect and support you.

VI. THE ENDING

11. END OF LIFE

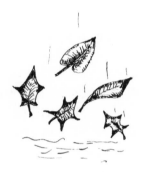

When I meet new patients who have come for a period of stay in the hospice, we talk about their journey: how they got to be in a hospice, about their experiences with their disease, and then we talk about the expectations from their stay. Around 50% of patients who are admitted do so for end-of-life care, to die. That means that 50% come in for control of troublesome symptoms, to then return home. When I meet patients at home who have a life-limiting illness it's no different. There are worries about what is coming and how it will feel. Patients say or ask similar things:

'Why am I here? I've come to die. It's my time and I'm fine about it.' **Edna 92,** who wasn't fine about it at all.

'I know it's daft, but how will you know I'm dead?' **Sandra, 44**

'I know I'm going to heaven, so I'm not frightened. Father Paul is praying for me.' **Janice, 83**

'I'm so frightened! Please hold my hand, tell me it'll be alright. I just don't want to know. Don't tell me. I've never cried in front of another man before. What's happening to me?' **Vik, 77**

'I'm fine today, thank you. I think I'll stay in bed and rest.' **Stefan, 66,** who went back to sleep and died later that day.

'I just want it to be over. I've had enough of carrying this around in me. It's too heavy now.' **Iréne, 73**

11.1 What usually happens when we die

One of the commonest fears we have is around the process of dying. Will you be in pain? Will you suffer? I try to reassure patients that their medical and social teams, alongside their loved ones, will aim to provide the care that they need, and that this will include control of any symptoms they are suffering.

I then check what kind of information they want: *'Is there anything in particular that worries you about dying, or that you need to know?'* Patients vary in their worries.

'Will I be cold?' **Agnes, 88**

'Will it hurt? I'm not afraid of pain.' **John, 68**

'I don't want to be alone!' **Ruth, 67**

'Will I choke?' **Ahmed, 44**

I reassure them that these things don't happen; it's not like that. Then I tell them that most deaths, no matter the diagnosis, tend to follow this similar pattern: you become less mobile, spending more and more time in bed. Alongside time in bed, there is increased tiredness and more time spent asleep. Your appetite lessens. You pass less urine. Hands and feet cool down and the circulatory system withdraws to the essential organs. You're semi-conscious now, responding to touch and questions but mostly asleep. Any pain or discomfort can be dealt with by medication. Otherwise there is a gradual drift to the end. Breathing changes, speeding up, slowing down, stopping, and then starting again. The desire for fluid lessens but it is still offered. Eventually breathing stops, then the heart stops, and then death has occurred. It is usually very peaceful. This process can occur over a matter of hours to days or even sometimes weeks. There isn't any hurry. We gather together and support you no matter how long it takes, and no matter what problems arise. We don't stop trying.

Even though you are sleepier, the team visiting you are skilled in assessing if you need more or less medication for any symptoms arising.

This pattern of gradual deterioration towards sleep and death is common, but it's not always like this. There are times when new symptoms arrive in the last days of life or old symptoms worsen. These can include pain, agitation and restlessness, noisy breathing and sometimes sickness. Most people get none of these, some get a little of one or the other and a few suffer from a greater degree of distress. The medical team aims to control any symptoms arising. They do this in a number of ways.

11.1i Treating physical symptoms in the last days and hours of life

Because swallowing becomes an issue at the end of life, medication, if used, can be given under the skin instead. Small pumps, called *syringe drivers*, deliver medication such as Morphine and anti-sickness drugs under the skin over a 24-hour period. The doses are checked regularly to ensure there is enough medication to provide comfort. Extra injections can be given if needed and these are called PRNs (Latin for Pro re nata, or As Required). Doses are also checked to make sure that you aren't receiving too much medication, which might add to any distress. If needed, and this is a rare occurrence, intravenous fluids can also be given under the skin for extra hydration rather than through a vein.

Pain, if pain has been a feature of the illness, can increase a little and a change in medication usually covers this. The commonest medications at this point are Morphine and Diamorphine, both of which can be given by injection rather than having to be swallowed.

Agitation is not uncommon at the end of life. To quote the Dylan Thomas poem, some people *'Do not go gently into that good night'*. The degree of agitation, like pain, is hugely variable. The medical team need to make sure there isn't a simple reason for this, such as a full bowel or bladder. If there is no obvious reversible cause then using sedative medication, usually a drug called Midazolam, reduces this distressing symptom and restlessness settles down. Rarely, agitation can become more of a feature. Another drug commonly used in this setting is Levomepromazine, a sedating drug that is also used for sickness. It is highly effective in providing calm once more.

Any nausea or vomiting can be controlled by making sure the patient is comfortable in bed, that they aren't constipated and that there isn't an infection – urine infections often cause nausea. If no reversible cause is found, medications can help to calm symptoms. Cancers commonly secrete substances that make us feel wretched. To treat nausea, common drugs like Cyclizine or Metoclopramide are used. There are quite a few other medications available too, in case these ones aren't effective.

Noisy 'wet' breathing can also occur, but isn't inevitable, at the end of life. Drugs used to dry this up include Hyoscine and Glycopyrronium. There is an adage in hospices that the noisy breathing is harder to listen to than for the patient to bear, as they are usually semi or unconscious by this time.

TIP: Please ask your doctor if you're concerned about what medication is being administered and what it is for.

Please rest assured that most people die in calm, undramatic ways. There is the occasional distressing death but these are rare. Please talk to your medical and spiritual team if you have particular concerns about what may happen to you. **In my experience most people die asleep, unaware of what is happening, drifting into an unknown oblivion.**

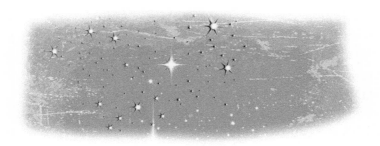

EXAMPLE 1

Kenny has had a tough time with his breathing. His COPD is in its final stages now, and the hospital feel there is no more they can offer. He came home with a Package of Care, oxygen, and an anxious nephew worrying about what was going to happen next. I went round on a home visit and spent some moments with Kenny before speaking to Ian:

'He's asleep all the time now. Not eating. Barely drinking. How's he going to keep his strength up?' asked Ian.

'Ian, what you're saying is what I would expect to happen. The time ahead for your uncle is very short now. It's natural for him to take less food and fluid. His body can't deal with it.'

'He gets really restless at night, too. Calling out.'

'I'm sorry to hear that. When did that last happen?'

'Couple of nights ago. Last night was OK, he slept through. But he gets shaky.'

'This all seems to in keeping with what I've seen before. I think your Uncle Kenny is now in the last days of his life.'

'I thought so.' Ian's voice cracks. *'I just want him to be OK. I want it to go away.'*

'It's really hard, isn't it? Is there anything in particular that you're worrying about?'

'Mm. What's going to happen?'

'You mean how will he die?'

'Yes, I suppose so. I've not seen it before. Dad went when I was little – it's why Uncle Kenny and I are so close – he's a bit like a father to me.'

There's a long pause. Ian looks out of the window. Then he turns to face me and shrugs. *'I don't know what to expect.'*

'I think it's going to be more of the same. More sleep, less drinking, drifting off quietly.'

'Can we turn off that oxygen? He pulls at the mask all the time.'

'Let me check.' Kenny grunts a little as I examine him but his eyes remain shut. I can barely rouse him. His oxygen levels are low but it feels to me that the mask is only causing a burden. It is unlikely to be making him comfortable any longer.

*'OK, let's take it off. Ian, I'm going to write up some medication for Kenny called anticipatory medication. It can be given for pain or restlessness. He won't necessarily need it, but if it's here, then we won't have to worry about it. If you see changes you are worried about, call the surgery for advice, if we're open, **and,** whatever the time, call the District Nurses, as they can give any necessary medication. I'll pop around tomorrow and see how you're both doing.'*

'OK, doctor. Thank you. See you tomorrow.'

After 24 hours, Kenny has deteriorated further. He has cool hands and feet, and his heart is beating quickly.

'How have things been?' I ask.

'Rough night. Uncle Kenny kept trying to get out of bed, pulling off the sheets. I called the District Nurses like you said, and they thought it was his bladder, that he needed a pee. I hadn't realised he'd not gone to the loo for hours. They put in a catheter and all this pee came out and I could see his face go all calm. He's been asleep ever since.'

'I'm glad they sorted it out. Yes, that can happen, when you feel too tired to get to the loo, but not sleepy enough to just let go in bed.'

'Uncle Kenny wouldn't have done that! He's so proud.'

'He seems really settled now. I'll call again tomorrow.'

'How long is this going to go on?'

*'I don't know. But I do know that you're doing a great job looking after him, and he looks really settled. Again, call us **and** the District Nurses if you need anything.'*

'Will do.'

That night, Kenny is agitated again, and the DNs go round to give some of the anticipatory medication.

'He went back to sleep,' Ian later tells me. *'He drifted off, looking like I'd never seen him, all drawn, but quiet. I brought Lucy in to sleep in her basket on this chair right by the bed. Thought that would be nice. I'm not sure if he noticed, but maybe he did... Anyway, he was so quiet, like I'd hoped. I fell asleep in the armchair, over there, and when I woke up... Uncle Kenny was gone.'*

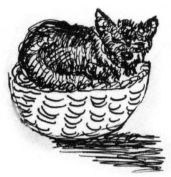

11.2 Where we choose to die

Most people continue to die in hospital rather than at home. Is this a bad thing? According to research, most people say they would like to spend their last days in their own homes. Not everyone wants to be at home, but knowing where you *would* like to spend your last days can help to improve the chances of achieving that goal.

For me, personally, it's really important to be at home, if possible, when my time comes. I want to be with my nearest and dearest and – like Kenny – my dog (she's called Elsie). I qualify this wish with the phrase *'if possible'*, because some circumstances may make my remaining at home untenable: I may become too frail, for instance, and require 24-hour nursing care, or develop difficult symptoms that would benefit from hospice admission. **Remember: hospices can care for people with ANY life-limiting illness, not just cancer.**

For some patients it's really important for them *not* to be at home. They worry about their loved ones taking on too many caring duties or not coping with the difficulties to come. Hospice can be an option if symptoms are difficult to control, or if someone is keen not to spend their last days at home.

Trying to pull this all together relies on knowing what you want and ensuring that there are services out there to provide those wishes. Even if you live on a farm, miles from a city, gathering information at times of serious illness helps teams to improve care and support wherever we are living, but it's best done as early on as possible, which is why we talked of it right at the start of this book, in Chapter 2.

There will also be times of crisis, when death in hospital can't be avoided even with the best-laid plans. It may also occur in the A&E department. The aim of medical teams in these settings is to ensure that good quality end-of-life care can be given, even in A&E. Wherever we die, hopefully the experience will be improved by good planning.

> **FACT: What we do know is that people's experience of end-of-life care is better if they are supported by a palliative care service.**

You also might like to bear in mind that research in the New England Journal of Medicine suggests that **people receiving best supportive care not only appear to suffer fewer symptoms, but may possibly even live longer than those undergoing more aggressive treatment**[47]. This research has not yet been replicated here in the UK, but it suggests aggressive treatment in terminal illness may not always be the best way forward, and this does tally with my experiences.

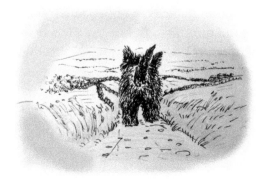

11.3 Unexpected endings – a note for family members

This is a troubling section to write. If you have worries about dying, then I'd suggest coming back to this section later – or skipping it altogether. It applies to very few people and you don't have to read it, please. It is more likely to be of help to your family if they have witnessed a troubling death than to you.

Though deaths at home and in the hospice are usually peaceful, there are some deaths that are less so. Despite medication to treat symptoms like pain or agitation, there are a rare few who do suffer in unexpected ways in their last hours.

This can be hard to anticipate. Sudden events like a bleed can occur. A large artery can leak, usually at the site of a tumour where tissue is fragile, and it can bleed a lot. This can happen in the skin, in the brain, in the lungs – anywhere. Remember, **IT'S REALLY UNCOMMON**. But if that one event happens to your loved one, it can be a hard thing to witness and the memory may haunt you. I would like to reassure you, dear reader, with this fact: large bleeds cause unconsciousness very quickly. Your loved one will be oblivious to the event within seconds. It will look messy as blood is a strongly staining material, but death comes swiftly and it will be over very quickly. If possible, medication can be given quickly to ease further any suffering but it happens so fast that often there isn't time to take action.

EXAMPLE 2

I was with Mike and his wife Carla when she died at the hospice. She had extensive endometrial cancer and was very frail. She had slipped into a coma, when out of the blue she started being sick. What came up was blood though, not vomit, and she appeared to wake up and then collapse back. It was over.

For Mike, the image of the blood was really upsetting. Despite Carla having had pain-free days of comfort and care, the last moments had left him with an image he couldn't resolve – was she aware in her final moments? Was she distressed? He felt responsible. It took weeks of counselling and reiteration that Carla would have known little of what had happened. Blood looks horrible, but the event lasted a couple of minutes at the most, and then she was gone.

At times like this I wish a spirit could return to tell us that everything was OK, that the person concerned felt only a moment of discomfort but wasn't really aware of what was happening. But my fantasy is for the rooms of clairvoyants. What I can offer is perspective: these more anguished deaths are **very rare** and the Palliative Care Team will have tried to anticipate as much as possible, but we can't anticipate every eventuality.

Mike eventually came to terms with what happened. After a year he stopped his sessions with the counsellor, and we heard he had met someone new and was going on a holiday with her. The way we scar over from these traumas doesn't mean they go away, rather we learn to live with them, another to add to the map of our own lives.

People with terminal diseases can also die of other causes, events that we can all die from every day. These can include heart attacks and clots on the lung called pulmonary embolisms (PEs). PEs can occur whilst walking, talking, or even sitting on the loo straining. Again, these unexpected events are quick and death usually arrives rapidly.

Because everything happens at speed, the frustration for relatives is commonly that they weren't present or couldn't get back in time. We can plan for a quiet, calm ending, and for everyone to be around, but that's not always going to happen. No matter how much we try, we can't control everything: as we said in Chapter 2, **no one ever knows exactly when they are going to die**. There are road accidents for humans just as there are for our beloved pets; the transition from health to dying can be momentary.

TIP: Perhaps consider this: rather than hanging onto the sad and upsetting moments at death, think instead about your last months and weeks which hopefully were more comfortable for your loved one. Moments together. Hold onto these memories, of last enjoyable weekends, treasured trips out, special times, and celebrations.

'*The last time I saw my father was on his 90th birthday. He was grumpy, overwhelmed and disengaged from the event. He died a few weeks later, relatively suddenly, and I wasn't there. But a few weeks before his birthday, I spent a couple of days looking after him when my stepmother was away and had a couple of friends round for the last evening. They're gay women and my dear dad thought one was a man – confusion was his middle name by this point – but no one was insulted; instead we all got very giggly and had a great evening. My friends were so patient with him even though he repeated the same questions, and when my friends left my dad insisted on coming to the front door and bellowing after them down the street, "I love you! I love you both!" I can't remember the actual last conversation I had with my father but this is the one I remember. My dad, filled with enthusiasm and love.*' **Sarah**

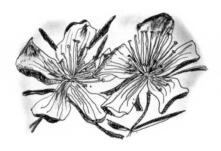

For your own notes:

....

....

....

....

....

....

....

....

....

....

....

....

....

....

....

....

12. YOUR LEGACY

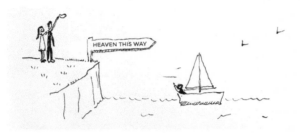

'I want to give everyone a glass of bubbly at the end of my funeral.'
Ira, 67

'It took us 10 years before we were all ready to scatter mum's ashes. We chose Sherwood Forest because we always walked there as kids. It's a place she loved, and we loved too.' **Isabella, 55**

Do you ever think about how you would like to be remembered, by family, friends and work colleagues? Some people are keen to engage in this, others find it too distressing. **It's worth considering the following pointers, perhaps as a way of prompting memories, and also ensuring that you are celebrated in the way that you wish.**

12.1 Memory boxes and life stories

We collect photos and letters and postcards and presents and cards in our lives. What do you do with yours? I keep mine in a particular box of treasured mementos. Not everything, just the ones that mean the most to me. These boxes of memory can help with recollections of good times and close moments.

People living with life-limiting illnesses who also have young families find that making a memory box for their child, who they won't be able to see grow up, helps to sort out their thoughts as well as focus on what is important to them[48]. Local hospices and Macmillan teams are adept at helping you to create these treasured memories. It's not just for those with children; we also use Memory Boxes for those losing their memory – dementia patients, whilst they're very much still alive – and anyone who would like to document their life, leaving a memento behind of who they were and what life meant to them.

My mother wrote me a short autobiography letting me know about her life before having children: growing up in Switzerland, memories of World War 2, life at school in the 1940s and her trip to England where she met my father. She described her family who lived abroad and about whom I knew little. This really helped me to understand more about her and to get a sense of my past.

There are no rules. Big or small, written memoirs or collected bits and pieces or both, it's up to you. You can include photos, letters, DVDs, treasured objects like jewellery, cards and even recipes, travel tickets, whatever it is that means something to you. The aim is to make something that celebrates your life, helping those that are left behind to remember you. It can be a kind of ritual making these boxes, a therapeutic gathering of thoughts and memories. It can be cathartic, helping to make sense of some of what's going on. For others it's too hard.

TIP: Take your time. Do what feels right for you.

12.2 Planning a funeral

I'm always amazed how organised people can be. They have their funeral paid for, the order of service written up and their favourite hymns chosen. Others, and I include myself, couldn't imagine doing this. For me, funerals are for those left behind, to celebrate in the way that they see fit. *'Some indication of what the person would have wanted can be helpful,'* says Sarah. *'My stepfather chose the hymns he wanted. I saw that as reflective of his thoughtfulness – giving us a steer gave us one less thing to worry about.'*

Each person is different; this is you and your loved ones' path to find. The route you follow can vary from a traditional funeral service in a sacred space, to a wilder option like an open-air rite in a forest.

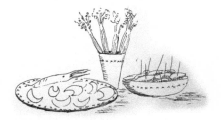

Here are some other things to consider:

- Religious or humanist – which is right for you? For some people, religion is central to their life, with a service at their local place of worship. For others it's important that there is no mention of God[49].
- Place of funeral – where would you like it to be? You're best advised to contact the relevant faith leader such as a priest, vicar, imam, rabbi or humanist celebrant[50].
- Flowers – or would you rather a donation to a charity? This is a common choice.
- Advertisement and death notice – often done in your local or national newspaper, you can say which.
- Travel to and from the service – organising transport is often done by the funeral director's team.
- Order of service – this can include readings, prayers, poems, songs, hymns, speeches from friends, quiet reflection time.
- Gathering after the service – what sort of place: pub, function room, at home? How much would you want to spend? Would it include refreshments?
- Rituals – what's important for those around you to know, from the lighting of candles to the recitation of a loved poem?
- Burial and headstone. What might an engraving say?

- Scattering of ashes – think about where this might be done, who with, and when.
- Anniversaries – marking the occasion annually.

12.3 Traditional or alternative?

Don't forget that there are alternatives to a regular funeral.

- Whilst tradition might lead you to organise a formal scattering or storage of ashes at a crematorium, perhaps with a tree or shrub planted in your honour, some people consider something called a **Natural Burial**[51]. For the ecologically minded there are also a variety of different ways forward, which you can explore on the Good Funeral website[52]. You'll see there are wide ranges of caskets that are very different from the traditional wooden kind – from sheep's wool to felt to willow baskets.

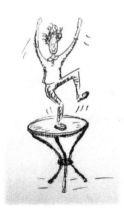

- **Celebrations.** For some, it feels that marking the end of a life should be a very solemn affair. For others, a more uplifting celebration feels fitting. Again, it can be whatever suits your situation and your passion. People have been known to ask for a party to be put on after their service, with balloons and cocktails.

- **Informal scatterings** are common too. Whether it is at a treasured location, at sea, in the woods, think about who should be there, and when would be the right time. There's no rush.

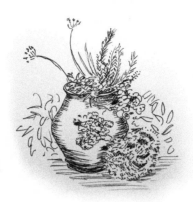

12.4 Financing a funeral

Funerals can be expensive (at the time of writing the average cost is around £3765[53]), so if your capacity for planning includes finances, you might consider a pre-paid scheme to ease any concerns you or your loved ones might have. Have a think about how much you would like to spend, and on what kind of service. *Which?* Magazine has some guidance[54] and there is more information about planning a funeral available via the links at the end of the book.

To have difficulty paying for a funeral is not that unusual. If you can't afford to pay for a funeral and there isn't the money in your estate to pay for it, the burden of payment can be declined by your family. Help is available via Social Services and also from charities such as Marie Curie. The amount contributed will go towards a service but it will be minimal. There are occasions when you can get a grant to help. The Palliative Care Social Worker should be able to help, or you can find suggestions at the back of the book[55].

If you are a named executor in the person's will, then the onus will be on you to organise payments from the estate but you won't be asked to pay out of your own pocket unless you are a family member.

TIP[56]: If you're concerned about budget and don't have strong feelings about having a burial spot, it's worth being aware that cremations are, on the whole, cheaper than burials.

If you would like to have your own DIY funeral this can be done, and it can also be done more cheaply. There is guidance online[57].

12.5 Memorials

In Italy there is a large cemetery outside the city of Genova called Staglieno. There are hundreds of very grand and elaborate headstones, sculptures, and chapels there. Acres of them. Photographs of the deceased adorn headstones. In America there are some graves with videos embedded in the headstones. In the Far East there are mausoleums built into the side of hills. Throughout the world we create memorials for those who have died. From a large Victorian sepulchre to a modest urn in the back garden, ultimately, all memorials serve the same purpose: to commemorate a life.

TIP: The Good Funeral Guide has some help and advice with organising memorials, whether it's a plaque on a park bench or a personalised engraving[58].

You might also want to think about a memorial ceremony as well as a funeral. This can be done anywhere, and with the celebrant of your choice, and if you leave it a while, it can mean your loved ones feel less emotionally raw, so if you are keen for them to celebrate, this might be a solution.

My family scattered our mum's ashes a year after her death in a field close to the home she had grown up in, miles away in Switzerland. We'd always known this was what she had wanted. We gathered together one September afternoon with a few of her close friends and it felt very personal and very fitting. Afterwards we all sat down to have lunch, swapping our memories of mum, sad and comical, toasting her memory, and giving thanks that we were all together to mark this special occasion.

From the simple to the lavish, there is a lot to think about, but if you've feelings about any of these issues, **please make your wishes known** as it will ease decisions for your relatives. Again, as with almost everything we've written in this book, it's a matter of choice and planning.

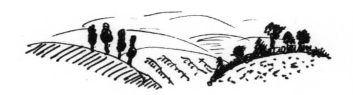

VII. FOR THOSE LEFT BEHIND

13. AND AFTERWARDS

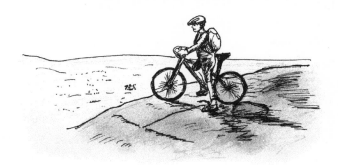

'I felt so numb after mum died, as if life had stopped. We went to register the death and, you know, I can't remember any of it. I'm slowly getting myself together now, but I miss her so much still.' **Jay, 44**

'He left us a letter to be read alongside the will. He went on about each of us, and how much we meant to him. I'll treasure that more than anything I've inherited and it made sorting out his affairs afterwards more of a pleasure, a way of honouring my dad.' **Lauren, 24**

After death, life continues for those left behind. Normal life can seem very weird, impossible even. How do we start picking up the pieces when all that we knew is no longer certain? What a grim time to have new responsibilities and decisions thrust on us. But the law has no feelings, and there are forms fill in, bills to pay and the world still spins. So let's have a brief look at what lies ahead for those bereaved.

13.1 Immediately after death

The body is there but the person has gone. Your loved one is no longer present; what remains is the container that they lived inside. The body will begin to cool down, the blood to congeal and the skin to contract.

There isn't a rush for relatives and loved ones to leave. Allow yourself to say goodbye, properly. **Take your time.**

If death happens at home, there should be a local protocol to follow. Firstly, a doctor or nurse is needed to verify that death has taken place. This will be the GP if the surgery is open, or the District Nurses if the surgery is shut. The DNs may call an Out-of-Hours GP for help. Avoid 999 as the ambulance crew are primed to try resuscitating someone unless a DNACPR form is in place as discussed in Chapter 11, and you won't wish for that to happen now. Verification is done by checking for the absence of breath and heart sounds. The body can then be released to the undertaker or taken into the local mortuary. Changes begin to occur to the body quickly but this can be slowed down by cooling. Any medical equipment is removed, including catheters, dressings and syringe drivers. The funeral director is contacted and they will take the body to their premises. They need to get the body into a cool place as soon as possible. The body is then cleaned and prepared.

If your usual doctor hasn't attended already, then they will be in touch to view the body and then to issue paperwork such as the medical cause of death certificate, which is discussed overleaf.

TIP: Now is the time to ask questions if you're troubled by anything that has happened or if there is anything that you haven't understood.

It's also a time for tears, for hugging, and for a new chapter of life to begin.

13.2 Post-mortems and the Coroner

If the *cause of death* is unclear, happens within 24 hours of hospital admission, or involves work-related circumstances (i.e. such as asbestos, or is unknown), then the Coroner's office are alerted. The Coroner's team will gather information from everyone involved in the patient's care including the family, aiming to establish a cause of death.

The Coroner may request a post-mortem – an examination of the body by a pathologist. The hospital team may also request a post-mortem if they are keen to know more about the disease process. There is more information about post-mortems on nhs.uk[59].

This may delay the funeral but the body is under the care of the Coroner's court until the Coroner releases it for funeral. It can also interfere with religious ceremonies, and it's important that any wishes and religious rituals[60] are highlighted to the court as early as possible.

After post-mortem, the Coroner holds a hearing or inquest to establish the cause of death. Evidence is considered, and then the coroner will give a verdict around the cause of death. They won't seek to apportion blame but the outcome of the court may have recommendations to take forward for those involved in the person's care. If you attend the Coroner's Court you will hear about your loved one's illness and their care. Some of this may be distressing but some of it may give you the information you need to better understand what has happened.

TIP: Don't attend the Coroner's Court alone. Have someone close come with you, for support and comfort.

If you have questions you want to ask, write them down in advance. If you feel something has gone wrong in your loved one's care, then you can highlight this to the Coroner, but remember the Coroner's role is purely to establish a cause of death, not to say who may be guilty of causing distress. The Coroner can refer on to the Prosecution Service if there is reason to consider foul play. There is supportive information and help from the Coroner's service on 0203 667 7884 or on the Coroner's Court website: coronerscourtssupportservice.org.uk.

13.3 Registration of Death

The family need to register the death. This is done by making an appointment with the Registrar of deaths at the local council offices and presenting the medical cause of death certificate that the doctor has provided. The Registrar will then issue a Death Certificate costing £12.50, and offer official copies at a cost, currently £4 per copy. Copies can then be used for insurance purposes. **Make sure that you ask for enough copies – at least two! Insurers, banks, credit agencies, etc, will all want an original copy. If you need further copies you can contact the Registrar's office but these will then cost £7.** All prices are for 2017.

If a cremation has been chosen, then there is further paperwork for doctors to complete. This requires a second doctor, who you won't know, to question those involved in the death to make sure there are no worries or concerns. The second doctor will speak to the doctor signing the first part of the form, who is your usual doctor, to the nursing team if they were involved, and to any family. Once completed, this form is reviewed by the cremation office doctor, and if all is in order then the process can commence.

13.4 Paying the bills

It's also at this time that the establishment becomes very unhelpful! Banks freeze assets, denying access to account until a death certificate is shown to them. Most funeral directors understand that there can be a delay in getting paid. Do let them know if this is the case. Bills continue to arrive, rent and mortgages need to be paid. There's a lot of sensible advice from the Money Advice Service[61]. The basic advice is:

- Notify the bank of any death as soon as possible.
- Notify the companies that supply services – gas, electrics, water.
- Notify the rental agency or landlord.
- Notify the mortgage holder.

But also think – who is the best person to be doing this? Is there anyone around to help?

13.5 Probate

A lawyer is next involved to issue probate. This establishes how the will is settled and how much money is owed to the government, how much in debts, and then to distribute the remainder to those who benefit from inheritance. If there is ONLY debt, then Social Services can help to sort out how to take financial matters forward. It would be best to speak to them as soon as possible, especially if bills are piling up.

Depending on how complicated the estate is, probate can be brief or it can go on for months. When my mum died, her very unhelpful solicitor dragged the process on for 18 months, partly because I didn't push hard enough and partly because they were lazy. Push them if you feel they are dragging their heels!

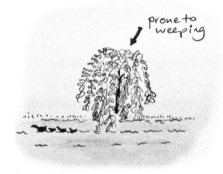
prone to weeping

13.6 As the days pass

Things change slowly for those left behind. Grief can be felt in a multitude of ways. Days pass into weeks, then six months, a year. There are anniversaries – birthdays, days of note in the illness of the previous year, other funerals to attend. Life continues as if nothing has happened. Many of us can cope with these changes, adapting to the loss, developing a scar inside us where our loved ones reside. We continue to talk to them, to imagine them with us and gradually this becomes a new kind of normal.

But for some people the grief is as sore as the first day of death. It is like a knife, cutting away, causing upset and tears, interfering with life. There doesn't seem to be a way forward. If after a few weeks you are feeling the same, as if the emptiness is as large and as painful as ever, then please seek support and help. Grief is a complex thing and support early on can make all the difference to recovery. This doesn't mean trying to forget what happened, or to forget the person who meant so much to you. Rather it's a matter of small steps. Of acknowledging the hole in your life and gradually building a new life around this. Mourning and grief will continue, why shouldn't it? But perhaps it won't be all-encompassing. Perhaps peace will come, step-by-step, day by day.

13.7 Last words

Dying, however long it takes, and some would argue it starts at birth, is a wildly various thing. Cultures differ, countries differ, even close neighbours differ on how they act and react to the changes within them. This book could never hope to be a thorough view of the passionate ways we live and die. But hopefully it has answered a few of the important questions around serious illness, and helped you to navigate the UK system of health and social care.

We both wish for you, and for all of us, a wonderful life, and a peaceful time in your dying and death.

Patrick and Sarah 2017

Note
We have aimed to be as thorough in our fact checking as possible but things still slip through despite sharp eyes. Do let us know if there is something important missing or wrong. Bear in mind that websites, correct today, may be absent tomorrow.

ACKNOWLEDGEMENTS

Patrick would like to thank:

Sarah, for the inspiration and the opportunity; Dr Rosemary Lennard and Dr Andrew Daley for igniting my interest in Palliative Care and giving me my first opportunity to do this work; Margaret Hayes, and all the astonishing Palliative Care Teams that I have worked with. Thanks too to the readers of early drafts for their feedback and support: Doreen O'Hara, Kathy Morton, Fern Smith, Philip Ralph and Claire Goad; to Laura Wilkinson and Mary Rayner for their help with the edits; to Leigh Forbes for the design. I am deeply indebted to Dr Rachel Sheils for reading and re-reading the manuscript, giving sage and pernickety advice, and for being an extraordinary sounding board at times of difficulty. Thanks to Karl and Elsie for tolerating me abandoning them to write this.

ENDNOTES

1. More information at sarah-rayner.com
2. There are statistics on life expectancy at the Office for National Statistics:
   https://www.ons.gov.uk/peoplepopulationandcommunity/birthsdeathsandmarriages/lifeexpectancies/bulletins/nationallifetablesunitedkingdom/2015-09-23
3. There are details on causes of death to be found here at the Office of Health Economics: www.ohe.org/publications/causes-death-study-century-change-england-and-wales. And here from the Office of National Statistics: visual.ons.gov.uk/what-are-the-top-causes-of-death-by-age-and-gender/.
4. A medical diagnosis is the process of determining which disease or condition explains a person's symptoms.
5. Gold Standards Framework (GSF) charity team:
   http://www.goldstandardsframework.org.uk/
6. NHS Advance Care Plan and Statement resources:
   http://www.nhs.uk/Planners/end-of-life-care/Pages/advance-statement.aspx
7. See also page 49: www.colostomyassociation.org.uk/index.php?
8. Marie Curie support:
   https://www.mariecurie.org.uk/help/support/being-there
9. https://www.nhsbsa.nhs.uk/help-travel-eye-care-wigs-and-fabric-support-costs/travel-receive-nhs-treatment
10. https://www.nhsbsa.nhs.uk/nhs-low-income-scheme
11. http://www.redcross.org.uk/What-we-do/Health-and-social-care/Independent-living/Transport-support
12. http://www.ncpc.org.uk/palliative-care-explained
13. You can see how this is done at this website:
    www.nhs.uk/Conditions/social-care-and-support-guide/Pages/assessment-care-needs.aspx#eligibility.
14. www.ageuk.org.uk/home-and-care/help-at-home/paying-for-care-and-support-at-home/
15. https://www.moneyadviceservice.org.uk/en/articles/are-you-eligible-for-nhs-continuing-care-funding
16. https://www.gov.uk/attendance-allowance/overview
17. www.ageuk.org.uk/home-and-care/care-homes/paying-for-permanent-residential-care/
18. https://www.alzheimers.org.uk/info/20030/staying_independent/201/keeping_safe_at_home/8

19. http://www.menopause.org/for-women/sexual-health-menopause-online/effective-treatments-for-sexual-problems/vaginal-and-vulvar-comfort-lubricants-moisturisers-and-low-dose-vaginal-estrogen.
20. www.blf.org.uk/your-stories/should-i-have-the-flu-jab).
21. Stages of grief: psychcentral.com/lib/the-5-stages-of-loss-and-grief/
22. See also *Making Friends with Your Fertility* by Tracey Sainsbury and Sarah Rayner.
23. https://patient.info/doctor/patient-health-questionnaire-phq-9
24. http://help.dyingmatters.org
    https://www.cruse.org.uk
    https://www.priorygroup.com/landing/fenchurch/bereavement-ppc
25. https://www.amazon.co.uk/Making-Friends-Anxiety-supportive-little-ebook/dp/B00N2R85QY
    https://www.amazon.co.uk/Making-Friends-Depression-companion-recovery-ebook/dp/B01LY27CMD/ref=pd_sim_351_3
26. http://www.henri-matisse.net/cut_outs.html
27. There's good advice from Macmillan here: http://www.macmillan.org.uk/information-and-support/organising/travel-and-holidays/travelling-abroad/taking-medicines-abroad.html
28. http://www.nhs.uk/conditions/tens/Pages/Introduction.aspx
29. gov.uk/make-will/overview
30. moneyadviceservice.org.uk/en/articles/diy-wills-what-you-need-to-know
31. There are details online about the MCA here: hra.nhs.uk/resources/research-legislation-and-governance/questions-and-answers-mental-capacity-act-2005/
32. There is more information about Best Interests meetings here: scie.org.uk/dementia/supporting-people-with-dementia/decisions/best-interest.asp
33. You can find out more about their role here: www.scie.org.uk/mca/imca
34. www.gov.uk/lasting-power-attorney-duties/health-welfare
35. ADRT information can be found here: www.nhs.uk/Planners/end-of-life-care/Pages/advance-decision-to-refuse-treatment.aspx
36. http://www.gmc-uk.org/guidance/28734.asp
37. www.macmillan.org.uk/information-and-support/organising/work-and-cancer/information-for-employees/your-rights.html
38. https://www.gov.uk/government/collections/fit-note
39. Phone number is 0808 8080000, www.macmillan.org.uk/information-and-support/organising/work-and-cancer/if-youre-self-employed/self-employment-and-cancer.html#161332
40. https://www.gov.uk/dismiss-staff/dismissals-due-to-illness
41. https://www.equalityadvisoryservice.com/ 0808 800 0082

42. https://www.moneyadviceservice.org.uk/en/articles/how-to-sort-out-your-money-if-you-become-ill-or-disabled
43. www.moneyadviceservice.org.uk/en/articles/dealing-with-the-debts-of-someone-who-has-died
44. www.moneyadviceservice.org.uk/en/tools/debt-advice-locator
45. https://www.gov.uk/attendance-allowance
46. https://www.citizensadvice.org.uk/benefits/sick-or-disabled-people-and-carers/pip/help-with-your-pip-claim/how-to-claim-if-terminally-ill/
47. http://www.nejm.org/doi/full/10.1056/NEJMoa1000678#t=article
48. The children's charity Winston's Wish has some ideas around this: https://www.winstonswish.org.uk/about-us/
49. https://humanism.org.uk/ceremonies/non-religious-funerals/
50. https://humanism.org.uk/ceremonies/find-a-celebrant/
51. http://www.naturaldeath.org.uk/index.php
52. http://www.goodfuneralguide.co.uk/find-a-funeral-director/what-is-a-green-funeral/ Author warning: there are graphic images on this site.
53. https://www.moneyadviceservice.org.uk/en/articles/how-much-does-a-funeral-cost#average-cost-of-a-funeral
54. More at their website: www.which.co.uk/money/insurance/funeral-plans/guides/funeral-plans-explained
55. https://www.moneyadviceservice.org.uk/en/articles/help-paying-for-a-funeral#what-happens-if-you-cant-afford-a-funeral https://www.mariecurie.org.uk/help/bereaved-family-friends/organising-funeral/funeral-payments http://www.qualitysolicitors.com/wills-and-probate/estate-administration/faq/who-is-responsible-for-arranging-and-paying-for-a-funeral
56. https://www.funeralzone.co.uk/help-resources/arranging-a-funeral/the-cost-of-a-funeral http://www.goodfuneralguide.co.uk/direct-disposal/ for cheaper option https://www.gov.uk/funeral-payments/what-youll-get for financial help, but it is often minimal.
57. http://www.goodfuneralguide.co.uk/find-a-funeral-director/do-it-all-yourself/ and here: http://www.naturaldeath.org.uk/index.php?page=book-shop
58. http://www.goodfuneralguide.co.uk/tombstones-and-ashes/marking-the-spot/
59. http://www.nhs.uk/conditions/Post-mortem/Pages/Introduction.aspx
60. Here is some helpful information on Muslim rites and post-mortems: http://www.mbcol.org.uk/funeral-procedure/h-m-coroner-and-post-mortem/#.WRmB-xMrKRs
61. The Money Advisory Service, who you can phone on 0800 138 7777 or view here: https://www.moneyadviceservice.org.uk/en/categories/when-someone-dies.

CHARITY CONTACT DETAILS
AND USEFUL WEBSITES

Here are the phone numbers and websites that you can find detailed throughout the book.

1. Discovering your own mortality
Causes of death:
- Office of National Statistics: ons.gov.uk/peoplepopulationand community/birthsdeathsandmarriages/lifeexpectancies/bulletins/nati onallifetablesunitedkingdom/2015-09-23
- visual.ons.gov.uk/what-are-the-top-causes-of-death-by-age-and-gender/
- Place of Death: endoflifecare-intelligence.org.uk/data_sources /place_of_death

2. Prognosis
- Advance Care Planning: nhs.uk/Planners/end-of-life-care/Pages/planning-ahead.aspx
- Gold Standards Framework: goldstandardsframework.org.uk/

3. Charity Contact Details
Macmillan Cancer Care provides a huge array of leaflets and support materials. It also gives information around cancer types as well as financial guidance. The phone line is currently open 9am - 8pm. The website offers chat rooms where patients can talk to each other about their experiences. This gives support and vital local information to new patients who in turn become the source of information in the future. There are lots of specific cancer charities too, including:

Cancer Care
- **Macmillan**, macmillan.org.uk **0808 808 0000**
- **Breast care**, breastcancercare.org.uk **0808 800 6000**
- **Prostate care**, prostatecanceruk.org **0800 074 8383**
- **Lymphoma care**, lymphomas.org.uk **0808 808 5555**
- **Lung Care**, blf.org.uk **03000 030 555**
- **Ovarian Care**, targetovariancancer.org.uk **020 7923 5475**
- **Bowel care**, beatingbowelcancer.org **020 8973 0011**

For more information around cancers and their treatments Cancer Research UK is a useful website: cancerresearchuk.org

Non-cancer Care
- **Heart failure**
British Heart Foundation, bhf.org.uk **0300 330 3311**
- **COPD:** British Lung Foundation, blf.org.uk **03000 030 555**
- **Renal failure**
Kidney Care UK, britishkidney-pa.co.uk **01420 541424**
- **Liver failure**:
Liver Trust, britishlivertrust.org.uk **0800 652 7330**
- **Parkinson's**: Parkinsons UK, parkinsons.org.uk **0808 800 0303**
- **Motor Neurone Disease**
MND Association, mndassociation.org **0808 802 6262**
- **Dementia**: Dementia UK, dementiauk.org **0800 888 6788**
- **Alzheimer's**: alzheimers.org.uk **0300 222 1122**
alz.org/uk/dementia-alzheimers-uk.asp
- **Progressive Supranuclear Palsy**
pspassociation.org.uk **0300 0110 122**
- **Stroke**: stroke.org.uk **0303 303 3100**
- **Multiple Sclerosis**
MS Society, mssociety.org.uk/what-is-ms **0808 800 8000**
- **Muscular dystrophy** **0800 652 6352**
musculardystrophyuk.org
- **Pulmonary Fibrosis**.................................. **no UK phone number**
www.pulmonaryfibrosis.org/life-with-pf/pulmonary-fibrosis-
treatment-options (American website)
- **Cystic Fibrosis**: cysticfibrosis.org.uk **0300 373 1000**
- **Colostomy UK**: colostomyuk.org **0800 328 4257**

General support
- **Age UK**: ageuk.org.uk **0800 169 2081**
This is the charity for older age. There will be a branch near you,
or if you live more remotely they have support on the phone.
- **Citizens Advice:** citizensadvice.org.uk **0345 404 0506**
Citizens Advice can help with support around the law and social care.
- **The Red Cross:** redcross.org.uk............................... **0344 871 1111**
We often think that The British Red Cross provide support abroad,
but they also provide help close to home. Their help is often needed
at times of crisis.
- **Carers UK:** carersuk.org **020 7378 4999**
- **Applying for travel finance help:**
  - nhsbsa.nhs.uk/help-travel-eye-care-wigs-and-fabric-support-
costs/travel-receive-nhs-treatment
  - nhsbsa.nhs.uk/nhs-low-income-schemeredcross.org.uk/What-
we-do/Health-and-social-care/Independent-living/Transport-
support

4. Wellbeing
- **Diets**
  - **Heart failure:** heart-failure.co.uk/living-with/lifestyle-changes/diet/index.htm
  - **Lung conditions:** www.blf.org.uk/support-for-you/eating-well/diet-and-my-symptoms
  - **Cancers:** macmillan.org.uk/information-and-support/coping/maintaining-a-healthy-lifestyle/healthy-eating
  - **Kidney disease:** www.kidney.org/nutrition
  - **Flu vaccine advice:** www.blf.org.uk/your-stories/should-i-have-the-flu-jab
- **Carers support:**
  - nhs.uk/Conditions/social-care-and-support-guide/Pages/assessment-care-needs.aspx#eligibility
  - ageuk.org.uk/home-and-care/help-at-home/paying-for-care-and-support-at-home/
  - ageuk.org.uk/home-and-care/care-homes/paying-for-permanent-residential-care/
  - mariecurie.org.uk/help/support/being-there
- **Women's sexual health:** menopause.org/for-women/sexual-health-menopause-online/effective-treatments-for-sexual-problems/vaginal-and-vulvar-comfort-lubricants-moisturizers-and-low-dose-vaginal-estrogen.
- **Assessing mood:** patient.info/doctor/patient-health-questionnaire-phq-9

5. Social Services and Benefits
- **Applying for benefits:** nhs.uk/Conditions/social-care-and-support-guide/Pages/assessment-care-needs.aspx#eligibility
- **Paying for support at home:** ageuk.org.uk/home-and-care/help-at-home/paying-for-care-and-support-at-home/
- **Funding Care:** moneyadviceservice.org.uk/en/articles/are-you-eligible-for-nhs-continuing-care-funding
- **Attendance Allowance:** https://www.gov.uk/attendance-allowance/overview
- **Residential Care:** www.ageuk.org.uk/home-and-care/care-homes/paying-for-permanent-residential-care/
- **Keeping safe at home:** www.alzheimers.org.uk/info/20030/staying_independent/201/keeping_safe_at_home/8
- **Travel advice:** www.macmillan.org.uk/information-and-support/organising/travel-and-holidays/travelling-abroad/taking-medicines-abroad.html

8. Medical Treatments
- **Assessing pain in Dementia:** eolp.co.uk/DEMENTIA/ images/Resources/Pain_assessment_2013_RCN.pdf
- **Treating pain** using the World Health Organisation ladder: www.who.int/cancer/palliative/painladder/en/
- **Continuing Health Care funding:** www.nhs.uk/Conditions/ social-care-and-support-guide/Pages/nhs-continuing-care.aspx
- **TENS Machines:** http://www.nhs.uk/conditions/tens/ Pages/Introduction.aspx

GP Computer Systems and Patient Access:
- **EMIS:** patient.emisaccess.co.uk/account/login?
- **VISION:** www.myvisiononline.co.uk/vpp/
- **SYSTMONE:** www.tpp-uk.com/products/systmonline

10. The Law
- **Wills:**
  - gov.uk/make-will/overview
  - moneyadviceservice.org.uk/en/articles/diy-wills-what-you-need-to-know
- **Mental Capacity Act:** hra.nhs.uk/resources/research-legislation-and-governance/questions-and-answers-mental-capacity-act-2005/
- **Power of attorney:**
  - www.gov.uk/power-of-attorney/overview
  - www.gov.uk/lasting-power-attorney-duties/property-financial-affairs.
  - www.gov.uk/lasting-power-attorney-duties/health-welfare
  - **Best Interests Meeting:** scie.org.uk/dementia/supporting-people-with-dementia/decisions/best-interest.asp
  - **Independent Mental Capacity Advocate:** www.scie.org.uk/mca/imca
- **Advance Care Planning:** www.nhs.uk/Planners/end-of-life-care/Pages/advance-decision-to-refuse-treatment.aspx
- **Resuscitation:**
  - www.resus.org.uk/faqs/faqs-cpr/
  - http://www.gmc-uk.org/guidance/28734.asp
  - **Advance Decisions to Refuse Treatment:** www.nhs.uk/Planners/end-of-life-care/Pages/advance-decision-to-refuse-treatment.aspx
- **Employment information**
  - **Your rights:** www.macmillan.org.uk/information-and-support/ organising/work-and-cancer/information-for-employees/your-rights.html
  - **Join a Union:** www.tuc.org.uk/join-union – how to join a union

- – **Sick notes:** www.gov.uk/government/collections/fit-note
- – **Discrimination at work:** Citizens Advice 0300 456 8390 http://www.citizensadvice.org.uk/
- – **Dismissal due to illness:** www.gov.uk/dismiss-staff/dismissals-due-to-illness
- – **Equality Advice:** https://www.equalityadvisoryservice.com/ 0808 800 0082
- – **Finances when ill:** www.moneyadviceservice.org.uk/en/articles/how-to-sort-out-your-money-if-you-become-ill-or-disabled
- **Sick Notes:** https://www.gov.uk/government/collections/fit-note

Debt
- – www.moneyadviceservice.org.uk/en/articles/dealing-with-the-debts-of-someone-who-has-died
- – **Locate Debt Advice:** www.moneyadviceservice.org.uk/en/tools/debt-advice-locator
- – **National Debtline** .... 0808 808 4000 www.nationaldebtline.org
- – **Step Change Debt Charity** .... 0800 138 1111 www.stepchange.org
- – **Debt Advice Foundation** .... 0800 622 6151 www.debtadvicefoundation.org

Benefits
- **Benefits checker:** citizensadvice.org.uk/benefits/benefits-introduction/what-benefits-can-i-get/benefit-checker/
- **Attendance Allowance:** gov.uk/attendance-allowance
- **PIPs:** citizensadvice.org.uk/benefits/sick-or-disabled-people-and-carers/pip/help-with-your-pip-claim/how-to-claim-if-terminally-ill/

Grants
- mariecurie.org.uk/help/benefits-entitlements/getting-help/grants
- macmillan.org.uk/information-and-support/organising/benefits-and-financial-support/benefits-and-your-rights/macmillan-grants.html
- mndassociation.org/getting-support/financial-support-information-for-people-with-mnd/

11. The Ending
- **Night sits**, Marie Curie ....0800 090 2309 www.mariecurie.org.uk/help/nursing-services

13. Afterwards
- **Funerals**
  - funeralzone.co.uk/help-resources/arranging-a-funeral/the-cost-of-a-funeral
  - goodfuneralguide.co.uk/direct-disposal/ for cheaper option
  - humanism.org.uk/ceremonies/find-a-celebrant/
  - naturaldeath.org.uk/index.php?page=find-a-natural-burial-site
  - goodfuneralguide.co.uk/find-a-funeral-director/what-is-a-green-funeral/

Paying for a funeral
- https://www.moneyadviceservice.org.uk/en/articles/how-much-does-a-funeral-cost#average-cost-of-a-funeral
- www.which.co.uk/money/insurance/funeral-plans/guides/funeral-plans-explained
- gov.uk/funeral-payments/what-youll-get
- www.moneyadviceservice.org.uk/en/articles/help-paying-for-a-funeral#what-happens-if-you-cant-afford-a-funeral
- https://www.mariecurie.org.uk/help/bereaved-family-friends/organising-funeral/funeral-payments
- http://www.qualitysolicitors.com/wills-and-probate/estate-administration/faq/who-is-responsible-for-arranging-and-paying-for-a-funeral
- http://www.goodfuneralguide.co.uk/find-a-funeral-director/do-it-all-yourself/
- http://www.naturaldeath.org.uk/index.php?page=book-shop

The Coroner
- **General Information:** **0203 667 7884**
  www.coronerscourtssupportservice.org.uk
- **Post Mortem:** http://www.nhs.uk/conditions/Post-mortem/Pages/Introduction.aspx
- **H.M. Coroner & Post Mortem:** www.mbcol.org.uk/funeral-procedure/h-m-coroner-and-post-mortem
- **When Someone Dies:** **0800 138 7777**
  www.moneyadviceservice.org.uk/en/categories/when-someone-dies.

Bereavement Support
- **Cruse Bereavement Care:** **0808 808 1677**
  crusebereavementcare.org.uk
- **Winston's Wish:** **01242 5151517**
  for help with Children's bereavement, winstonswish.org.uk/about-us/
- priorygroup.com/landing/fenchurch/bereavement-ppc

Memorials

- goodfuneralguide.co.uk/tombstones-and-ashes/marking-the-spot/
- humanism.org.uk/ceremonies/non-religious-funerals
- which.co.uk/money/insurance/funeral-plans/guides/funeral-plans-explained
- goodfuneralguide.co.uk/find-a-funeral-director/what-is-a-green-funeral/
- deadgoodguides.co.uk: a website dedicated to designing your own funeral and courses on how to be a celebrant.
- greenfuse.co.uk: a website dedicated to training celebrants and undertakers

RECOMMENDED READING

Here are some of our favourite books on the subject of ageing, palliation, dying and grief.

On Mortality by Atul Gawande.
This is a seminal work, and we would encourage anyone who is interested in this subject to read it.

On Death and Dying by Elizabeth Kübler-Ross.
Another seminal work, examining the stages of grieving.

Mortality by Christopher Hitchens.
A darkly funny book about living with a terminal illness, by the caustic journalist.

The Conversation by Angelo Volandes.
A plea for better palliative care in America.

When Breath Becomes Air by Paul Kalinithi.
A personal reflection on a doctor's own diagnosis of a terminal illness.

Dancing With Mister D: Notes on Life and Death by Bert Keizer.
A personal experience of caring for the terminally ill.

A Very Easy Death by Simone de Beauvoir.

Tuesdays with Morrie by Mitch Albom.

Nothing to be Frightened of by Julian Barnes.

Benedictus: A Book of Blessings by John O'Donohue.
A beautiful book of celebratory poetry for every occasion.

Intimate Death: How The Dying Teach Us To Live by Carol Brown Janeway and Marie De Hennezel.

The American Way of Death by Jessica Mitford.
A tale of funeral directors and their strange business.

The End of Life Advisor by Susan Dolan.
Detailed support and advice for those in the USA.

The End of Life Handbook by David B Feldman and S. Andrew Lasher. Offers support and advice for those in the USA. Unravelling the American medical system and a plea for advance decision to be made by everyone.

The Oxford Textbook of Palliative Care Edited by Nathan Cherny (Editor), Marie Fallon (Editor), Stein Kaasa (Editor), Russell K. Portenoy (Editor), David C. Currow (Editor).
The standard medical textbook now in its 5th edition.

Palliative Care Formulary (PCF) by Robert Twycross and Andrew Wilcock. A comprehensive guide to medication used in End of Life Care

Friends have also recommended the following memoirs:
Dying by Cory Taylor
The Iceberg by Marion Coutts
The Year of Magical Thinking by Joan Didion
A Grief Observed by C.S. Lewis

There are also lots of books on chemotherapy and radiotherapy. There are more on living well with your illness and coping with disease and its burdens. We passionately believe that getting good quality information helps make the journey ahead easier – please take some time looking for the right material for you.

Making Friends with Anxiety:
A warm, supportive little book to help ease worry and panic

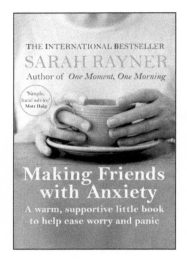

'Simple, lucid advice on how to accept your anxiety' **Matt Haig, bestselling author of *Reasons to Stay Alive.***

Drawing on her experience of **anxiety disorder and recovery**, Sarah Rayner explores this common and often distressing condition with candour and humour. She reveals **the seven elements that commonly contribute to anxiety** including adrenaline, negative thinking and fear of the future, and explains why it becomes such a problem for many of us. **Packed with tips and exercises** and offset by the author's photographs and anecdotes from her life, if you suffer from panic attacks, a debilitating disorder or just want to reduce the amount of time you spend worrying, *Making Friends with Anxiety* will give you a greater understanding of how your mind and body work together, helping restore confidence and control.

- Uses **Mindfulness-based Cognitive Therapy** techniques
- Includes **photographs** by the author to lift the spirit
- **Useful links** throughout, plus details of **helplines** and **recommended reads**
- Online support available – share experiences and tips with over 7000 members

'Reads like chatting with an old friend; one with wit, wisdom and experience' **Laura Lockington, Brighton and Hove Independent**

Making Friends with the Menopause:
A clear and comforting guide to support you as your body changes
2017 edition reflecting the new 'NICE' guidelines

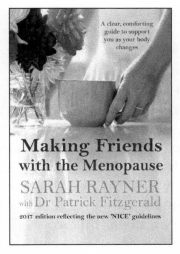

Written with Sarah Rayner's trademark warmth and humour, this **new edition of the popular *Making Friends with the Menopause* has been updated to reflect the latest National Institute for Health and Care guidelines on diagnosis and management of the menopause**. Together with Dr Patrick Fitzgerald, she explores why stopping menstruating causes such profound chemical changes in the body, leading us to react in a myriad of ways physically and mentally. There is practical advice on hot flushes and night sweats, anxiety and mood swings, muscular aches and loss of libido, early-onset menopause, hysterectomy and more, plus a simple explanation of each stage of the menopause so you'll know what to expect. You'll find details of the treatment options available, together with tips and insights from women keen to share their wisdom. Whether you're worried about feeling invisible, weight gain or loss of fertility, or simply want to take care of yourself well, knowledge is power, and *Making Friends with the Menopause* will give you a greater understanding of the process, so you can enjoy your body and your sexuality as you age.

- Includes advice on all the major health issues that can arise as a result of hormone change
- Includes traditional and complementary medicine
- Gives guidance on how to get the most from your GP appointments and finding good alternative practitioners
- Useful links throughout, plus details of helplines and recommended reads

Making Friends with Depression:
A warm and wise companion to recovery

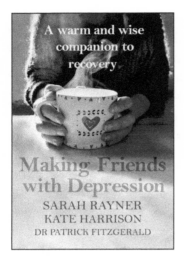

From the bestselling authors of *Making Friends with Anxiety* and *The 5/2 Diet Book* comes a clear and comforting book to help sufferers of depression.

If you're suffering very low mood, you can end up feeling very alone, desperately struggling to find a way through, but recovery *is* possible and Sarah Rayner and Kate Harrison, together with Dr Patrick Fitzgerald show you how. They explain that hating or fighting the 'black dog' of depression can actually prolong your suffering, whereas 'making friends' with your darker emotions by compassionately accepting these feelings can restore health and happiness.

Sarah and Kate write with candour, compassion and humour because they've both been there and, together with Dr Patrick Fitzgerald, have produced a concise and practical guide to help lift low mood and support the journey to recovery. It explains:

- The different types of depressive illness
- Where to seek help and how to get a diagnosis
- The pros and cons of the most common medications
- The different kinds of therapy available
- Why depression can cause so many physical symptoms… and much more.

Making Friends with Your Fertility
A clear and comforting guide to reproductive health

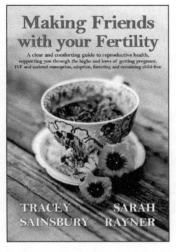

'A must read… A robust, resilient friend for everyone considering their fertility and an essential addition to any fertility professional's bookshelf' **Susan Seenan, Chief Executive, Fertility Network UK**

From the onset of periods and puberty, through egg and sperm production and preparing to conceive naturally, to IVF and assisted conception, in *Making Friends with your Fertility*, counsellor Tracey Sainsbury and bestselling author Sarah Rayner them all with warmth and humour. Together they take you on a journey not just exploring what happens when things go well (through intercourse, orgasm and pregnancy), but also looking at situations where conception is not so straightforward, as it isn't for 1 in 6 heterosexual couples experiencing infertility or for those who are single or in same sex relationships and keen to have a baby. And *Making Friends with your Fertility* is not just for those trying to conceive – it's for all those keen to support them – friends and family, counsellors and healthcare professionals too.

The result is a handy, practical primer that makes these complex and sometimes distressing issues less confusing and overwhelming, supporting each individual with sensitivity and honesty so they can 'make friends' with their own fertility, in whatever form that takes.

Making Peace with Divorce

A warm, supportive guide to separating and starting anew

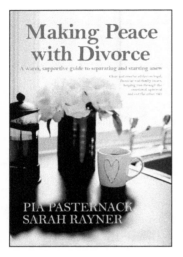

After 20 years of marriage and three children, full-time mum Pia Pasternack came home one day to find a note on the doormat and her husband gone...

Heartbroken, this was the first of a series of revelations that left her and her family reeling. But gradually Pia built herself back up, and in *Making Peace with Divorce*, written together with best-selling author Sarah Rayner (*Making Friends with Anxiety, One Moment, One Morning*) Pia passes on the lessons she has learned about the legal, financial and emotional implications of separation.

Together they guide you through the minefield that accompanies the bust-up of many long-term relationships, explor-ing with warmth and humour sensitive issues such as whether to separate, how to break the news to children (if you have them) and how best to communicate with your ex. You'll find clear and concise guidance on finding a lawyer, filling in forms and reaching a settlement. And if a settlement cannot be reached, there's the low-down to help prepare you for what happens at court.

There are quick tips to aid your own recovery, insights from others from all walks of life who have been through separation, and pointers on how to move on. The result is a handy, practical and uplifting guide that will make this distressing time less confusing and overwhelming, supporting you so you can 'make peace' with your own divorce or separation, thereby creating a happy and fulfilling future.

One Moment, One Morning: A novel

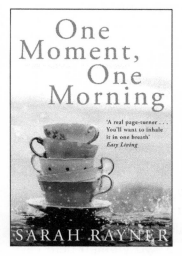

'Carried along by the momentum of a suspense-filled yet touching story that drives to the core of human emotion, this book is a real page-turner, exploring the harrowing pain of loss and grief, family secrets and how a tragic event can force you to be honest about who you really are. A real page-turner . . . You'll want to inhale it in one breath'.
Easy Living

The Brighton to London line. The 07:44 train. Carriages packed with commuters. A woman applies her make-up. Another occupies her time observing the people around her. A husband and wife share an affectionate gesture. Further along, a woman flicks through a glossy magazine. Then, abruptly, everything changes: a man has a heart attack, and can't be resuscitated; the train is stopped, an ambulance called. For three passengers on the 07:44 that particular morning, life will never be the same again.

'Touching, insightful, this is a story that will stay with you'.
Take a Break Fiction Feast

'An intimate, thoughtful novel celebrating women's friendship and loyalty.'
Waterstone's Books Quarterly

The Two Week Wait: A novel

What if the thing you most longed for was resting on a two week wait?

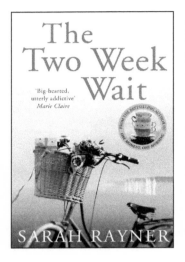

After a health scare, Brighton-based Lou learns that her time to have a baby is running out. She can't imagine a future without children, but her partner, Sofia, doesn't seem to feel the same way.

Meanwhile, up in Yorkshire, Cath is longing to start a family with her husband, Rich. No one would be happier to have a child than Rich, but Cath is infertile.

Could these two women help each other out?

'A topical subject treated with insightfulness and care; a wholly absorbing story will prompt a tear or two'. **Easy Living**

'In evoking ordinary lives invaded by a deep, primitive yearning, Rayner's portrayal of her characters interior landscapes is carefully crafted and empathetic'. **The Sunday Times**

'Incredibly compelling... Beautifully written and heartbreakingly honest.' **Novelicious**

Another Night, Another Day: A novel

Three people, each crying out for help . . .

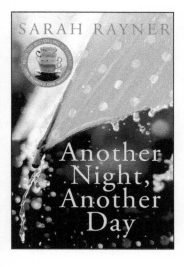

There's Karen, worried about her dying father; Abby, whose son has autism and needs constant care; and Michael, a family man on the verge of bankruptcy. As each sinks under the strain, they're brought together at Moreland's Clinic. Here, behind closed doors, they reveal their deepest secrets, confront and console one another and share plenty of laughs. But how will they cope when a new crisis strikes?

'Written from the heart' **The Bookseller**

'I was engaged and moved by this irresistible novel about friendship, family and dealing with life's blows'. **Woman & Home**

'Brilliant ... Warm and approachable, with fascinating characters.'
Essentials

'Powerful ... A sympathetic insight into the causes and effects of mental ill-health as they affect ordinary people.' **My Weekly**